Do No Harm

The Story of a Doctor's Vision and Practice Of Humanitarian Medicine

By

Yoshitaka Ohno, M.D., Ph.D.

© 2000, 2001 by Dr. Yoshitaka Ohno. All rights reserved.

No part of this book may be reproduced, stored in a retrieval system, or transmitted by any means, electronic, mechanical, photocopying, recording, or otherwise, without written permission from the author.

ISBN: 0-75964-053-X

This book is printed on acid free paper.

1stBooks – rev. 10/8/01

"I will apply dietetic measures for the benefit of the sick according to my ability and judgment; I will keep them from harm and injustice".

From the Hippocratic Oath, Fifth Century B.C.

During this same time, Hippocrates suspected a connection between disease and environment, and stated:

"One should consider attentively the waters which inhabitants use."

I wonder what Hippocrates would say if he were alive today?

Dedication

To Akiko, my wife. It is to you that I dedicate this book with my deepest love. I also dedicate this book to the forces of the universe and to my ancestors, who guided me to such a wonderful woman.

With Deepest Gratitude

There are many people whom I wish to extend my appreciation, because without their support and faith in me this book would not have been possible. I first want to thank my mother, Yoshiko Ohno. From the time I can remember, my mother has always told me how important it is for me to be a humanitarian doctor. Her love and unending trust has enabled me to establish the Ohno Institute, which is not mine alone, but devoted to anyone who will benefit from it. Her faith in me transcends the miles from Japan to America, where I feel her sending her strength to me. Without her, I would never have had the fortitude to write this book.

I also wish to honor the memories of my ancestors, especially my father, Yoshio Ohno, my grandfather, Ryozo Ohno, and my grandmother, Mikino Ohno. I always feel their energy reaching me from their eternal rest. I can always hear them telling me, "Taka, we are always watching over you! Never worry about your future because we will always help and protect you. Always try to accomplish your best, that is all we want from you. We are very proud of you and we send our praise for your efforts. Be happy, Taka. We love you!" I believe in the energy of my ancestors and I honor their spirits in everything I do.

I appreciate and honor my uncle, Dr. Yoriaki Hamuro, who is the chief priest at Kasuga Taisha Shrine, in Nara Japan. He has always encouraged me with his strong spiritual energy, which has given me a tremendous amount of insight about my personal path. Thank you, Uncle, for being such a wonderful role model. I hope I can continue to follow in your footsteps and, like you, be an inspiration for many people who turn to me for help and guidance.

I want to thank my older brother, Dr. Yoshioki Ohno, president of the Ohno Hospital in Osaka, Japan. Because he is dedicated to running our hospital, I am able to live in America and to pursue my work. I also want to extend my gratitude to him for successfully operating on our mother and saving her life from breast cancer. Yoshioki is a gifted doctor and surgeon, and I am very proud to be his brother.

I want to thank my cousin, Shigeyuki Torigoe who handles my business affairs in Japan. I can feel confident that Shigeyuki is managing effectively with his kind heart and an honesty, which is coupled with his strong business knowledge.

I wish to thank my father-in-law, Dr. Yoshihiko Tsubura who has been like a father to me. Dr. Tsubura helped me enter the Nara Medical University, where he gave me the unique opportunity to perform special research on cancer, which enabled me to obtain a Ph.D. He has been a true role model as he has taught me by example the importance of being a humanitarian doctor.

In addition to my family, many fellow doctors have given me their love and support. I also wish to thank my patients, who have given me their complete trust.

Without them I would not have been able to conduct my many studies. I owe my patients a tremendous amount of gratitude for their faith in my work.

I also want to express my appreciation to Loni Chiarella for her sensitivity in capturing the feeling of my message in editing this book, as well as her role as my personal advisor. I am very grateful for her encouragement and her patience.

I want to extend my gratitude for the staff of the Ohno Institute, who support my efforts on a daily level. May you all continue to grow with me in the years to come.

I especially want to thank Dr. Howard Reminick, my friend and associate who helped me build the Institute, for carefully reviewing and doing the final edit.

Finally, I give my heartfelt appreciation to my beloved wife, Akiko, as well as my much loved children, Ayako, Naoko and Fumitaka. Since the day we married, Akiko has supported me completely. I would definitely not be where I am today if it weren't for her. Since we have been married, we have never quarreled. Akiko is a true lady in every sense of the word. When I have gone through difficult times of internal struggle, she has always given me sound advice to help me conquer my difficulties. Even though we have gone through many tough times since we have been married, she has never complained because her trust in me is beyond measure.

I am a typical Japanese man, so I am always devoted to my work and my study. There are times when I take no time off, no Sundays, or holidays. However, Akiko has never complained about my work because she knows how important it is to me. Even when I don't get home until after midnight, Akiko will always have a wonderful dinner prepared for me. If she were not my wife, my life would have been completely different. She is not only my wife, but also my best friend.

Preface

Sometimes it takes the effort of reflecting on the collective experience of many years to make us realize that the moment of defeat was really the beginning of our victory. It is true; my life has been a succession of many painful experiences. But as I reflect upon each crisis, I recognize that as I have progressed through every event, there has also been a new part of me that has awakened. My inner being has always emerged in a positive way, gradually making me a more centered and focused person. And as I have evolved and become more balanced and spiritually connected, my life has given rise to a new level of commitment.

This book is about the times in my life when I had to encounter many struggles in order to gain understanding and have appreciation of the final outcome. While I report the horrors I experienced during my years of practicing medicine in Japan, I also show how I gradually found a way to answer the cries of despair for my patients. This was not easy. It required that I make a decision that would put me at professional risk and force me to leave my practice. But during this process of change, I learned to become a better doctor, more concerned about the welfare of my patients, than the rewards of fame and fortune, which, unfortunately, has become modern medicine.

I did not have to take this road. It would have been easier to follow the program and do what I was told to do by my superiors. I come from a very prominent family. I have always had choices and opportunities. But the values given to me by my family led to the decision to take actions, which, though distressing at first, brought me to what I believe is my destiny. Without the experiences during this journey, I would have never been receptive to receive and understand the vision that was given to me, a vision that brings hope to anyone seeking a better, longer and fuller life.

During this journey I gained insight and learned to view my life with new understanding. I found the place where the seeds of knowledge are formed. I also found answers to how each of us is able to take some control of how we want to live the rest of our lives. This is how I received the message, which was to become my vision, a vision that weaves its way throughout the story of my journey.

I believe that there has always been an invisible force within me guiding my direction and encouraging me to discover my true calling in life. As I have proceeded through this transformation, there is one principal factor that has continually surfaced and risen to the top. This factor above all else has captured my awareness and remains today a focus in my life. The factor is contribution, the act of giving to others, directly from one's heart. This affects not only the recipients of our gestures, but of equal importance, the essence of our personal being.

I also believe, more than anything else, that my vision to help humanity is derived directly from giving people the awareness of how vitally important contribution is to the soul of the benefactor. My vision has become a vehicle that can assist people to gain an understanding that as they direct their energies to give of themselves with a pure and open heart, they will ultimately fill an emptiness that resides deep within their spiritual center.

My book encompasses the actual journey I experienced in my own personal search in discovering the importance of contribution. There is a saying that it is not until someone has lived through a particular experience that they are able to develop empathy that is needed to help others in similar situations. For this I am grateful.

My destiny has taken the shape of my personal contribution to help humanity through the vision, which I call Shintopia; a mind, body and spirit healing unity and its connection to a philosophy of living with gratitude and respect for nature. It is based on the wisdom of ancient healing arts, together with sound scientific, medical knowledge. By practicing and teaching this

Shintopian vision, many people with whom I have had contact now enjoy a healthier and fuller life.

Through years of study and experimentation, I found the significant interrelationship of health and nature, and its impact on the quality of life. The best example is our precious water supply. After you read this book, you should become more knowledgeable about how the quality of the water in our body can be the difference between health and sickness. You should also understand why it is imperative to redirect our priorities and efforts to take better care of our limited water sources. You will also understand why it is crucial to have the best water possible available for human consumption, so we can enjoy a healthier, longer and fuller life.

In 1997, I founded the Ohno Institute on Water and Health, a non-profit organization, to foster research, education, training, and the dissemination of the information on chronic and aging disorders. The focus of the work at the Institute is to study and promote the benefits of the naturally magnetized water I discovered in Japan, which has been shown to have a major effect in preventing diseases associated with aging, as well as delaying the aging process.

Early in my career, I began to search for ways to stop the suffering of my patients who had degenerative diseases such as cancer, Alzheimer's, multiple sclerosis; and diseases such as hypertension, asthma and diabetes, which needed to be managed with constant medications. I realized that the side effects of these medications were creating serious problems, and increasing the body's deterioration. After further study, I became convinced that the condition of the body's water was related to the way the body continually deteriorated and recovered from disease.

In order to test this theory, I studied and tested many water sources. While I was conducting research in Japan, I discovered naturally magnetized water that was being used by a prominent physician with his patients suffering from the same diseases. As I observed and studied these patients, it became apparent that this water was unique and had therapeutic benefits. To prevent this gift from being exploited, I purchased the mountain and the water rights, and I have made it my life's mission to distribute this very special water to as many people as I possibly can. It is through making this water available to people that my vision of a way to a healthier, fuller and longer life will ultimately be made known.

I invite you to accompany me for awhile as I reflect upon my life's work and passion. As you live with me through the experiences which I describe in this book, you should be able to comprehend the essence and the total meaning of my Shintopian vision, which has helped me fulfill my mother's wish that I become a humanitarian doctor.

Table of Contents

		Page
Chapter 1	The Rude Awakening	1
Chapter 2	My Personal Transformation	18
Chapter 3	The Maruyama Vaccine	33
Chapter 4	The Healing Process Continues at Nara Medical Hospital	49
Chapter 5	Destiny Awakening	64
Chapter 6	Returning Home	83
Chapter 7	The Living Waters of Japan's Ancient Magnetic Mountain	101
Chapter 8	Bringing Japan's Gift of Life to America	120
Chapter 9	Sharing My Vision	136

Chapter One

The Rude Awakening
University Hospital, Osaka Japan

Our painful experiences become the passages that open our hearts to empathy.

"Please help me die, Dr. Ohno! Please help me die! I know you can help me, Dr. Ohno. Please show mercy and help me! Stop this pain I am going through! I beg of you, Dr. Ohno, be merciful and help me die. Send me to heaven and relieve me of my pain!"

She stunned me with her outburst. I responded. "I know you are in a state of intense pain and you are not able to think straight! Please understand that what you ask of me is unthinkable and I cannot help you die. I am a doctor!"

She took deep and deliberate breaths. It was obvious that she was in a tremendous amount of pain because of the anticancer medication in her system. I wondered if it was the pain that had taken over her senses, affecting her sanity. But her eyes told me that she was not insane, quite the opposite. In fact, she was quite rational, and her intention was very clear.

"Dr. Ohno, please understand, I am asking you to do this out of mercy for me! I am asking the 'unthinkable' because you are my doctor, and I trust that you will help me. If you were not my doctor, and if I felt you did not care for me, I would never think of requesting such a thing.

"I have been waiting for the right time to approach you. I have been praying to God to give me the chance to talk to you. It is at this moment that I am telling you that I have decided to die. I have hesitated because I knew, of course, how you would react to my request. Your reaction is not a surprise to me. I would not have expected you to react in any other way!"

Yoshitaka Ohno, M.D., Ph.D.

She looked at me carefully and calmly. She was almost too calm. She had surrendered herself totally to this decision. There was no fear in her voice or in her eyes. She was resolved in her conviction to die. She got up out of her bed and closed the door quietly, wanting privacy in the room so no one else would hear our conversation.

"Dr. Ohno, I have asked you before to stop giving me the anticancer drug! The side effects are too strong and I know you don't want to watch me suffer! Every time you inject me with this drug, I know you, too, are suffering as you watch me suffer.

"I have lost over 25 pounds since I have been here. I weighed 100 pounds when I was first admitted and now I weigh only 75 pounds. Look at me! I look like a living skeleton! Nobody recognizes me anymore, because I am only a shadow of the person I used to be!

"Putting food into my mouth is a nightmare because I know I will vomit up everything I eat. When there is no food in my stomach, then I experience the dry heaves. Right now I am also suffering from bleeding of my gums. It looks like I never clean or brush my teeth."

Her eyes were filling with tears again. She suddenly held her hand out from underneath her bed sheet and said, "Look! Look at my finger!" When she showed me her finger, I noticed that the fingernail had fallen off and the skin under the nail had turned black.

"Look at my finger. It looks like a dead person's!" She waved her finger in front of me to see. Sobbing, she lifted off her wig. "My hair has completely fallen out! I am completely bald! I can tolerate my hair loss, but I have no energy left to stand the continuous nausea and vomiting and chills! The chills that take over my body after you inject me with the anticancer drug are terrible. It doesn't matter how many blankets I use to cover myself with, the chills are so intense that nothing makes me warm!

"After the chills subside, I have another severe attack of abdominal pain. The pain is so strong that I have to take another

Do No Harm

drug to ease the pain. After the abdominal cramps, I can't move my arms or legs. When I go to pick up something, I have no feeling. Even if I prick myself with a needle, I am numb and feel nothing. After the paralysis, I have nausea again with more vomiting.

"Dr. Ohno, even though I am a strong and patient person, I cannot tolerate these strong side effects. I am reaching the end of my limit! Dr. Ohno, I beg of you, please stop giving me the anticancer drug! I have experienced strong side effects before from anticancer drugs, but this new anticancer drug has worse side effects. They are unbearable for me to tolerate. I know I do not have the strength to handle the pain anymore!"

Her words lingered in the room, hovering over me like a thick, dark cloud. It was very clear that she was nearing the end of her pain tolerance. She was getting weaker every time I saw her. Her voice was very strained now. Simple conversation was very difficult for her. But she found energy to make an appeal to me.

I sat there in the room with her, struggling for something to say. At that moment, there was nothing I could tell her, no words I could find to say to her, to give her any comfort. Although I felt compassion for her, a part of me wanted to get up and leave the room. I wanted to process what was happening, not only to her, but to me as well. Just as I thought of leaving the room, she instinctively reached over and grabbed my hand. I remember how the strength in her frail and lifeless hand amazed me. I felt the inner strength of her soul at that moment. As I hesitated, searching for a way to bring comfort to her, she continued…

" Dr Ohno… from the first time I met you, and looked into your caring eyes, I knew you were a person who would understand. I sensed that you were completely different from the other doctors who had treated me before. I felt this way because I watched how truly sincere and empathic you were with your patients.

Yoshitaka Ohno, M.D., Ph.D.

"The other doctors have always ignored me while I have struggled with the agony of my pain. But your eyes have always shown me your genuine concern. I have never found another doctor who has demonstrated compassion the way you do.

"I am aware that you do not agree with the hospital professor and you want to stop giving me the anticancer drug. I know that you suffer from being embarrassed about this situation and that you are deeply troubled because of your disagreement with the professor on how I should be treated. I know that if it were up to you, you would be taking care of me in a completely different way."

Again, her statement caught me totally by surprise, I responded, "What?" I suddenly raised my voice to her. "How do you know such things? Who has spoken to you about this?"

She reached over and gently patted my hand. It seemed so strange to watch her comfort me while I was searching for a way to bring comfort to her. Then she said, "No one has had to tell me anything. I know of your personal struggle because your face is always pale and drawn. I have been watching you and I have recognized your personal battle. Your work is depressing and you are aging and looking older and tired from the struggle."

She was talking to me with concern in her voice as though I were her son. Her insights were amazingly accurate. She stopped and took a sip of tea. During the silence, I started thinking about what she had just said.

It was true that I was struggling and my physical state was showing the fatigue from my internal battle. I was not sleeping well. I would not go to bed until after 1:00 in the morning every night. As tired as I was, I would lie in my bed unable to sleep. Since I could not sleep, I would usually get up and sit at my desk. I would think about her and if there were possibly different ways of helping her. I often thought to myself, "*Why did I become a doctor?*"

When I first became a doctor, I thought that I would find ways to help my patients. But instead of a healer, I felt more like a murderer. I was aware that the struggle would continue for me

Do No Harm

if I didn't find a better way to help my patients. I realized that I must decide whether I could continue being a doctor. I knew I would not remain the kind of doctor who could not effectively care for his patients. Nearly every night I would lose sleep over my preoccupation with this concern. During the day, my eyes were red and weary from lack of proper sleep, and I was being emotionally drained.

She finished her tea and continued, "Since I have been here, I have become very fond of you because you remind me of my son. I always think to myself that if I die, Dr. Ohno will be with me at my deathbed. This thought gives me a feeling of comfort.

"I have tried my best to be a good patient. I have never complained or refused your help because I have believed in you with all of my being. I have trusted you with my life. However, I cannot tolerate taking this new anticancer drug anymore, because the side effects are too strong for me to handle."

She held my hands and looked directly into my eyes. Then she continued to speak....

"I have talked to my family about my decision to ask you to help me die. I have made them promise me that they will not see you or bother you after my death. I am trying to make this easy for you to do. All I want you to do is to put another drug in the tube. That is all you have to do and then walk away. Or, you can just leave the drug on the table and I will pick it up and swallow it. You can leave the room and leave me to die in peace and my pain will be over. If you are a humanitarian doctor, you will obey your patient's last wish. You are the only doctor who can help me! My family will not blame you; they will be appreciative because they know of my wish to die.

"Please send me to heaven right now! "Please, Dr. Ohno, please send me to heaven!"

She was convulsing and weeping. Her frail and lifeless body shook with her sobs. I immediately answered, "I cannot help you die! I am a doctor, not a murderer! I have taken an oath to help keep people alive. I know you are in a tremendous amount of pain, but I cannot help you die!

Yoshitaka Ohno, M.D., Ph.D.

"Please don't ask me again! I cannot help you. Not in that way!"

A part of me died that day, watching this woman collapsing in sobs and begging me to release her from her misery. This incident I just described happened shortly after I graduated from medical school and was interning in Orthopedics at the University of Osaka, in Osaka, Japan. When I first met her, she was a 62-year-old breast cancer patient, being treated in the outpatient clinic. I saw her husband first and I thought he was my patient because he looked as though he had no energy, and he was so thin.

The nurse accompanied the couple into the examination room. When they entered the room I realized that I had misunderstood who the patient was. I asked her to give me a brief description of her medical history and she began,

"I was found to have breast cancer five years ago. I was operated on at a different hospital and at first, it seemed that the operation had been successful and that all the cancer had been removed. However, one year after the operation, the cancer reappeared again, so I was put on the anticancer drug. The anticancer drug worked for awhile, but then the cancer reappeared.

"The last doctor I had did not care about terminally ill cancer patients. The doctor and his staff encouraged me to be discharged from the hospital and they suggested that I go to hospice. I do not want to go to hospice because I have not lost my will to live. I have decided to fight the cancer and fight for my life!

"This is why I have come to your hospital."

As she talked about the details of her breast cancer, her X rays were delivered to the examination room. As I reviewed her x-rays, I was shocked to see that the cancer had metastasized to her pelvis and to her brain. I thought to myself, *it is impossible to help her at this stage of the cancer. All she can do now is try to be as comfortable as possible and wait for her inevitable death.*

Do No Harm

Then I spoke to her as honestly and kindly as I could. "Your cancer has already metastasized to your pelvic bone. And it has also metastasized to your brain.

"Unfortunately, I am also recommending that you go to the hospice because we can do nothing for you now. It is too late to try alternative measures because your cancer has already spread to the extent that there is no therapy that can help you at the stage of your cancer. The damage is irreversible.

"I realize this sounds cruel to you, but the more chemotherapy you are given, the sooner you will die. You see, the anticancer drug kills not only cancer cells in your body, but destroys even healthy cells. It cannot distinguish between a cancerous cell and a healthy cell. As a result healthy cells are destroyed. Your body loses its immune ability and death results soon afterward.

"The anticancer drug is generally successful when only a small part of the body has been affected by cancer. But your case is a completely different situation because the cancer has spread throughout your body.

"I don't recommend chemotherapy because it is too hard on patients. The side effects are too strong and counteract what the chemotherapy is designed to do. I suggest that you should consider an alternative measure."

Objecting to my recommendations, she said, "It doesn't matter to me what the painful side effects are from the anticancer drug, because I have to get well so that I can take care of my husband! That is why I will keep trying to fight the cancer!

"Please admit me right now so that you can begin to help me! If I go to the hospice, then I am surrendering myself to death. I refuse to surrender my life until I know within my heart that I have no choice!"

"I know how difficult this must be for you and I do understand how you must feel, but right now our hospital is full. Even if there was something we could do for you, we don't have a bed for you at this time. Please understand that although I wish

Yoshitaka Ohno, M.D., Ph.D.

I could, there is nothing that I can do to help you. I am suggesting that you go home."

"No! I can't go home! My husband is not healthy. He is very weak and I need to look after him. If something were to happen to me, he would surely die very soon because he is not able to care for himself.

"Please, Dr. Ohno, admit me into the hospital now! Please find a way, any way, to cure my cancer!"

The scene in the clinic was a heartbreaking one. This sweet and loving couple had obviously been together and devoted to one another for many years. Although she was literally dying from the cancer that had taken over her body, she was more concerned in her husband and her responsibility to take care of him. I so desperately wanted to be able to give them both some kind of hope. But the facts were in the X-rays, and there wasn't anything I could do at this point in time to help her.

"As I have already told you, the hospital is full. If you decide you want to come back, you will need to wait until we have the room to admit you."

"You don't understand, Dr.Ohno! I don't have time! I only have now and I need a miracle! Please reconsider and admit me! Can't you make a special provision for me, because I am an end-stage cancer patient?"

At that moment, the hospital medical professor, who was my superior, stepped into the examination room and interrupted the conversation. "Dr. Ohno, I will take care of this patient. I will be able to help her. You should take care of another patient."

He continued, "I am sorry to interrupt your conversation. Let me introduce myself, I am the main professor of the hospital. My name is Doctor 'A'.

"I have had the opportunity to look at your X rays. Because your cancer has metastasized to your pelvic bone and to your brain, I agree with Dr. Ohno that it is not going to be easy at this stage of your cancer. The cure rate is only five percent for end-stage cancer, and unfortunately in your case, I don't see any hope."

Do No Harm

He watched her face intently. The color in her face turned completely pale. He waited for the impact of the news for her chances of survival to set in. Once he saw the couple's reaction and how discouraged she and her husband were, he then continued, "I think I can save you with a new drug I have developed.

"This new drug only destroys the cancer cells and it has no side effects, based upon animal testing. It is true that this drug is in the experimental stages, but the data from the testing has shown that there is a definite decline in the cancer, as well as showing not to have any side effects. I can offer you this opportunity for a possible cure for your cancer!

"This new anticancer drug has never been used in another hospital. If more cancer patients knew about this special drug, the response would be tremendous! You are very fortunate that you have come to our hospital and met me."

The professor's words were totally unexpected by her. Her expression changed from one of despair to an expression of hope. She and her husband began to cry with tears of joy and relief.

She grasped the professor's hand and said, "Oh, thank you so very much! I never expected a miracle like this from your hospital! You have given me hope again!"

The couple held each other and cried from the good news. The scene touched everyone in the room. The professor was very pleased with himself. As I watched this dramatic scene, it seemed as though I were watching a scene out of a movie. However, despite the deep emotion of the event that had just taken place, I felt completely separated from the joy that everyone else was experiencing. I knew that the anticancer drug the professor was talking about absolutely had very strong side effects.

I wondered why the professor insisted on using the anticancer drug on this woman. I internally questioned his decision and I felt very uncomfortable for this patient because I suspected that his recommendation was not in the patient's best interest.

This was the first of what was to prove to be many rude awakenings for me. After years of medical school, of learning how to help people, I was now coming face to face with the grim reality of obeying a hospital staff professor, who was treating patients as though they were experimental animals. There was no empathy for people who were terminally ill. I wanted desperately to disagree with him, but I was only an intern.

The Japanese medical system is very conservative. The professors on staff are upheld as though they were royalty, and the interns are looked upon as nothing more than slaves. I knew if I said anything to question him I would probably be fired on the spot.

The professor ordered the breast cancer patient to be admitted into our hospital. Immediately after being admitted, she received the anticancer drug twice a week. Then a course of agony began for this patient. The new anticancer drug had devastating side effects. It took hold of its victim with a force so intense that the agony of the pain was unbearable.

"Please stop giving me this drug, Dr. Ohno, I beg of you! Please help to take the pain in my stomach away! The professor told me that there would be no side effects from this drug and I am in agony!"

"Please stop this pain! Please stop it!"

The tragedy of this scene would repeat itself over and over, becoming my ongoing personal nightmare. The anticancer drug was given to the patient, and after each injection her life energy to withstand the trauma declined. Even though I knew I was not responsible for causing her pain, I was in fact the doctor who administered the injection. I watched as other interns around me were able to go about their daily routine. I noticed that they were able to set themselves apart from the pain their patients were experiencing. However, this was impossible for me to do.

I felt so much empathy for my patients that it was very difficult for me to stand by and do nothing, especially when I

Do No Harm

knew in my heart that some of these patients were not receiving the right kind of care. But again, I kept reminding myself that I was only an intern and perhaps this was something I needed to work through so that I could eventually become the kind of doctor I knew I could be. I was determined to become a doctor who healed people and a doctor who was able to make a positive change in people's lives.

Yoshitaka Ohno, M.D., Ph.D.

Torn

There are times in our life that we experience the internal crossroads of doing what feels right in our heart and what external pressures expect us to do.
These challenges aid us in the development of our character

"No! You are not amputating my hand! I will never allow you to cut off my hand! I need both of my hands! Please, please tell me that you are not going to cut off my hand!"

Silence, tears, and screams... she was in a state of disbelief and terrorized by the thought of amputation.

"If you want to take my hand, you'll have to wait until after I am dead! I am not some experimental animal.

"Please, Dr. Ohno! Tell them not to amputate my hand! Please, please, I beg of you!"

This is a tragic story that I experienced at the same hospital three years later. She was a very young and talented girl with such a kind and friendly personality. She attracted many people, and everyone wanted to be her friend. She was not only the promising star of her gymnastics team, but she was also a beauty with the heart of an angel. She was as intelligent as she was lovely. Her parents had high hopes that she would enter medical school and become a doctor someday. She mastered all of her subjects in school with high honors. Everything in her future seemed bright and promising. No one could ever imagine that death was lingering beside her like a terrible, dark shadow.

One day after she turned 15 years old, she began to feel a swelling and a hot spot in her shoulder. At first she thought this was caused by an insect bite so she ignored it. However, the discomfort continued for over a month. She never complained about the symptoms to her parents or her gymnastics coach. She was concentrating on her gymnastics competition that was soon to take place, and she didn't want to concern anyone needlessly.

Do No Harm

Although she continued to feel the pain, she ignored it, hoping it would eventually subside.

Then, her bright future came to a halt. It all became apparent during gymnastics practice, when in the middle of doing a routine cartwheel, she experienced a severe pain in her shoulder. She ignored the pain and continued to practice another cartwheel. This time the pain intensified and she felt a very strange 'crack' inside her shoulder. The pain became severe. It literally took away her breath. She fell to the floor in excruciating pain, screaming, "Someone help me! I think... I think I broke my arm!"

Within moments she fell to the floor unconscious from the pain. Her gymnastics coach and her friends immediately surrounded her.

"Call an ambulance! Someone, quickly call an ambulance!"

The gymnastics coach then said, "No one move her! Wait until the ambulance arrives. We don't want to take a chance and cause more damage to her shoulder!"

Off and on she would awaken, scream out again in pain, and fall suddenly back into an unconscious state.

At the hospital, her X-rays were read by the emergency room doctor, who told her, "Your humerus bone has been fractured. There is also a mass showing up in your X-rays and I feel we should take a closer look at it. I suggest that we admit you into the hospital for a biopsy as soon as possible."

The next day the biopsy was taken and sent to the pathology department for analysis. When the doctor received the results from the biopsy, he went to the young girl and her family and reviewed the results of her biopsy. They watched as the doctor opened the envelope containing the pathology report. As his eyes scanned the report, the look on his face dramatically changed and he became very somber. After what seemed like an eternity, he read the results to the young girl and her family.

"I am sorry to say that I have some very bad news. The pathologist's report shows a tumor on the humerus."

Yoshitaka Ohno, M.D., Ph.D.

Everyone was quiet for a moment. Her father asked, "Is the tumor benign... or malignant?"

"The tumor is malignant." The doctor added, "It is so far advanced that if we performed an operation to remove the tumor, her chance of living for five years would only be 20 percent. The X rays also indicate that the cancer has already metastasized to the lung."

Her parents wept upon hearing the devastating news. The young girl's eyes filled with tears, but she held her emotions. Upon hearing the news, the young girl and her parents went to another hospital to seek a second opinion. Unfortunately, the prognosis was the same. They then proceeded to go to three more hospitals. The prognosis from all the hospitals was virtually the same. Finally, they returned to the University Hospital.

I was among the staff present when the young girl and her parents heard the recommendation from the professor, "We should amputate her arm from the shoulder immediately. We need to perform the amputation as soon as possible, in order to increase her chance of survival."

The young girl responded emphatically, "No! This is *my* body! *My* arm! *My* life! It's not your life! I will not consider amputating my arm, and I don't care what the consequences are!"

There was a long discussion between the girl, her parents and the professor over the amputation. The tension in the room was strong as the professor attempted to persuade her to have the amputation. Her parents believed that if she went through with the amputation, it would help prolong her life. But the young girl was emphatic about her decision to not go through with the procedure.

"After I die you can amputate my arm for the tests you want to perform, but I will not allow the amputation while I am alive! Even though my mother is crying and trying to persuade me, I cannot agree with her. This is my body, not

Do No Harm

my mother's body. I am 15 years old and I will decide what is best for my body and my life!"

One last time, the professor very sternly told her, "You should have the amputation and it has to be done immediately. If you do not go through with the amputation you will surely die very soon. You must reconsider!"

Once again, I was internally questioning the opinion of the professor. I knew that her cancer had already metastasized to her lung and there was nothing that amputating her arm would do to help her live longer. I wondered why he was so emphatic about recommending the amputation.

I later realized that the professor wanted to perform the amputation because her tumor was very rare. If the amputation were to be done while the girl was still alive, the tumor would also be alive. The live tumor was necessary for his personal experimental research.

The professor continued to pressure her to have the amputation. However, she still refused. The professor and her family finally gave up. Then the professor offered his only alternative, the new anticancer drug.

The days to follow would present me with a similar scene of watching a patient in torment, as I would again be called upon to administer the anticancer drug to the young girl. Once again, I was obeying an order from the professor. An order to give a patient a painful drug that went against my personal and professional judgment. I struggled emotionally and mentally, moment by moment, torn between what I was expected to do and what I knew was the right thing to do.

Three days after I had started injecting the anticancer drug into the young girl, the nightmare of her agony took hold. She had no appetite; she experienced ongoing nausea and vomiting. The fatigue from fighting her suffering was overwhelming.

"Please, Dr. Ohno, please don't give me any more injections! I can't take the pain of the side effects anymore!

My stomach feels like it's pushing its way up through my mouth. I've had so many seizures!

"Please make this hell stop! Please! Stop giving me this drug!"

She was completely fatigued. She was collapsing and sobbing. I watched as her face turned pale from the effects of the drug. I witnessed her tough and fighting spirit fade into a lifeless agony.

She had huge sores in her mouth from the side effects of the drug. The sores were so bad she could not swallow, let alone eat. The seizures were intensifying. It was becoming more difficult for her to breathe. Compounding her misery were other side effects of chronic headaches, fever and infection. Medicine to help eliminate these was not working.

"Help me Dr. Ohno! I have already lost 20 pounds! I cannot eat anything, because nothing stays in my stomach. No one has any idea how much I am suffering! Please stop giving me that drug! I know I am dying. I don't want to take this drug anymore!"

If the positive benefits had offset the negative side effects, I might have been more understanding and less resistant. But this was not the case. I began to feel that this drug was a monster. I felt that I was not a doctor, but I was being forced against my better judgment to administer this 'Devil's Drug' which was torturing and killing my patients! I would ask myself, "Am I really a doctor, or am I just a prisoner of the medical system?"

Question after question kept entering my mind, *How can I stop giving my patients this horrible drug when I know it is torturing them? How can I stand by and allow myself to remain a part of this if I know it is wrong? How can I continue to call myself a doctor when I think of myself as a killer?*

I knew for my own preservation and peace of mind that I had to do something else to help my patients. I decided to commit myself to finding another way to help these people, and hopefully by doing so, I would heal myself of the personal torment I was living through.

*Struggle can be a blessing in disguise.
There is no room to grow if the Universe does not present challenges.*

Yoshitaka Ohno, M.D., Ph.D.

Chapter Two

My Personal Transformation

*Nothing exists in our consciousness unless
we allow it to be there.
We have the power to create change –
Anytime we decide to do so.*

During the time I was watching my breast cancer and bone tumor patients fight for their survival, I was deeply aware that I, too, was fighting for the survival of my personal integrity. I was in the midst of a major crossroads that would ultimately affect the direction of my life. My patients were the catalysts that would create a testing ground for me to either make the choices that would honor my personal truth or cause me to fall in with the mass of followers. I could not be one of those who do not listen to the voice of their conscience, but take the safe road to achieve their goals.

Through my internship at University Hospital, I made long-lasting friendships with other interns. I would talk with the interns I was closest to about the anticancer drug and how it affected the patients. I expressed my doubts about the continued use of this 'Devil's Drug' and that I believed I needed to stop giving it to the patients. We had many discussions about whether these feelings were right or wrong. I shared with them that I felt more like a killer than a doctor. But time and time again, the answers from the other interns were always the same. They seemed to echo in unison,

"The hospital professor is very powerful! If you disagree with him and do not follow his orders and give the anticancer drug to patients as you are instructed, he will become very angry. You will never be able to receive your Ph.D. at this hospital! You will have to go somewhere else."

Do No Harm

"We should always obey what is asked of us. This is the only way we can become doctors and go on for our Ph.D.s. We cannot argue with what we are told, or we will be fired and lose all hope for our future in the medical field!"

I remembered one story told to me that happened at this hospital. It happened long before I arrived. There was a doctor on the staff, a good doctor and a kind person. He was a humanitarian doctor. He was always concerned for his patients. He was not like some of the other doctors, only interested in their careers and their future, such as becoming a professor or making more money. He disliked prescribing drugs, even though his professor insisted. It troubled him to watch his cancer patients suffer from the overuse of drugs, especially the new experimental anticancer drugs. Instead, he would use alternative therapies that he believed were safer and more natural. Because he did not follow his professor's orders, he was fired.

Even though he was a good doctor with a good reputation, he could not find another position because his professor used his influence with other hospitals. He became so frustrated and disgusted that he quit medicine.

The Japanese medical society is an elite class. It respects and takes care of doctors from universities with the most reputation and power. They are the only ones who ever become professors in prestigious hospitals. Those who graduate and are trained at other, less prestigious universities have a difficult time getting opportunities to practice at prestigious hospitals. If a doctor is a graduate of the same medical school as his medical superior, he will be treated differently.

Under the strong power and influence of a professor, hospitals can get doctors to fill their staff. The president or director of a hospital will go to the professor and request doctors. How they show respect and patronize the professor will determine if they are successful.

Because my family has a long history in medicine and owns a large, successful hospital in Osaka, Japan, other doctors have treated me with jealousy. When I decided that my patients were

Yoshitaka Ohno, M.D., Ph.D.

being given too much of a dangerous drug and decreased the amount of dose, another doctor would change my order on the patient's chart and raise the dose without notifying me.

Knowing that I would never be able to respect my professor or the doctors who jumped to his orders, I had to make a career decision before I lost my desire to continue to practice medicine. Besides turning to fellow interns who were my friends for advice, I turned to my family for advice as well. I respected the wisdom of my mother, who had tremendous insight and heart. She, without a doubt has had the largest impact in my life. Her words of wisdom would ring loud and clear within my soul. Ultimately, it would be her influence that would lead me through my struggle and toward the destiny I didn't at the time understand.

The turning point in my life that enabled me to come to terms with my own personal truth were the words I heard her speak to me when I was only 16 years of age.

"What I would like to say to you is that you should never be a 'money' doctor. If you will be a doctor who is focused on money, your life will be short because of resentment. However, if you become a humanitarian doctor, your life will be so full of happiness and you, as well as the people who you help, will be forever grateful."

These are the words my mother said to me on the day my father died. Because of the untimely death of my father at such a young age, and the circumstances surrounding his death, my mother's words will remain with me forever.

My family's tragedy
1963

What happened to my father?
He was such a healthy person!
I can't believe he is gone today when just yesterday he was so healthy!

Do No Harm

Why had we not noticed the situation of his ailing health in time?

Especially since my father was a doctor, why was he not able to tell us that he had not been feeling well?

Why was modern medicine not able to prevent his stroke?

I couldn't believe he was gone. I feared for our future and wondered if we would ever be able to have a normal life again.

My father died when he was just 42 years old. He was a very famous surgeon whose specialty was cancer surgery. He had a tremendous amount of drive and energy. He started and developed the Ohno Hospital in Osaka, Japan into a very renowned institution. He was driven to become the president of the Japan Medical Society. He was an exceptionally hard worker and never believed in taking a break. He went to the hospital every day to see his patients, even on Saturday and Sunday. The only time he took a day off was on New Year's Day.

His main interest was pancreatic cancer, and he had a research center in the hospital so that he could continue his search for a cure. After he finished his daily schedule of surgery, he would always go to the research center to study until midnight. There were times he would stay longer if he was performing an animal experiment. I rarely saw him and I would ask my mother why he was not home. She answered, "Father has stayed at the research center to finish his experiment."

December 8, 1963, was a cold winter's day with the forecast of snow. I was just 16 years old. That morning when I woke up, my father was still home. To see him home at this hour was very strange, because he always left for the hospital very early in the morning. He was never home for me to see him when I got ready for school.

"Good morning, Father!" I said.

He did not answer me immediately because he was not feeling well. I wasn't aware at the time that he was in physical pain so I ignored his delayed response and didn't think very

Yoshitaka Ohno, M.D., Ph.D.

much of it at that moment. Seeing him home that winter morning is the last memory I have of seeing my father alive.

As soon as he arrived at the hospital that morning, he asked a nurse to check his blood pressure. The nurse took his blood pressure and said,

"Dr. Ohno! You're blood pressure is dangerously high! Your blood pressure is exceptionally high and the reading is 220/120! It is impossible for you to perform the surgery you have scheduled today!"

"Please cancel today's surgery because your own health is in a very serious situation! Dr. Ohno, I am very concerned that you will suffer a heart attack or a stroke! Please stop your plans to operate!"

Very quickly my father firmly instructed the nurse to be quiet and insisted that she not tell anyone about his high blood pressure.

"Don't worry about my blood pressure!" he said. "I am strong and healthy and I won't have a stroke! Don't worry about my health. You must keep quiet about this matter. After I am finished with the surgery today, I will take a break and relax."

When he went into the operating room, he began to feel dizzy and it was not easy for him to stand. He ignored his symptoms because he never for a moment believed he would actually have a stroke! When he continued to prepare for the operation, he felt nauseous and light headed while washing his hands. His head was pounding with excruciating pain and he felt that he must have been having a migraine headache.

He had never experienced so much pain in all of his life. The thought of stopping the operation finally entered his mind, but when he looked around he saw that everything was prepared for the surgical procedure for the esophagus cancer patient. The doctors, nurses, all of the instruments and the patient was prepped and waiting for him to begin. He denied his thought to stop the operation but decided that he definitely would take a break right after he was through with the procedure.

Do No Harm

But the opportunity for him to take a break never came. After he began the operation his conditions worsened and his face started to turn pale. One of the nurses recognized the lack of color in his face and said, "Dr. Ohno! Your face is very pale! You need to take a break! Let somebody take your place today!"

He wiped the perspiration from his brow and said, "Don't worry, I am all right. I can do this operation. Don't worry about my body, please concentrate on the patient and the procedure instead!"

The nurse hesitated for a moment said, "I understand."

However, thirty minutes into the operation, he began to experience a severe pain. "I cannot tolerate this headache! Please, help me! Please help me!"

But once the operation had started the other doctors and nurses could not stop the procedure. Again he shouted out, "Please, help me stop this headache!

Please…stop this headache!"

When he screamed these words, he suddenly fell to the floor and lost all consciousness. He was having a stroke.

As this was happening, I was at school when someone came into my class and asked for me. "Is there a Yoshitaka Ohno in this class?"

I raised my hand and said "Yes, I am here. What is wrong, has something happened?"

He said, "You should go to the Ohno Hospital immediately! Your father has taken ill and your mother has sent for you! You need to leave right now!"

"What?" I said to him.

I couldn't understand what he had told me because my father was such a healthy person. I hoped this was a misunderstanding, but as I closely studied his face, I knew it was true. I started to feel like I would break down once I realized what had happened.

Then my teacher shouted, "Yoshitaka! You should go to the hospital right now! This is very serious. We have sent for a taxi to take you to the hospital, so prepare yourself to leave immediately!"

Yoshitaka Ohno, M.D., Ph.D.

I picked up my school bag and went to the taxi. I was in a daze during the ride to the hospital. Over and over in my mind I was thinking that even though they had said that my father's condition was very serious, I couldn't bring myself to believe it was true. He was such a healthy man. I imagined him living until he was 120 years old! Just last night he had bought "sushi" and brought it home for us. Perhaps someone had made a terrible mistake. Perhaps it was someone else. Perhaps the teacher had made a mistake. Maybe it was my grandfather who had taken ill. I believed that this was a mistake and I had gotten the wrong news.

However, when I arrived at the hospital, my hopes were crushed completely when I talked to the nurse and realized that it was true. It was not my grandfather or someone else, it was indeed my father who was ill.

The nurse said to me, "Your father is in a coma. He is not doing well, even though we had the best surgeons operate on him. His situation is very grave because he had a stroke and the large blood vessel in his brain ruptured."

"I want to go to his room and see him right now!" I told her.

She said, " You can't see him because he is in recovery. You need to go to the waiting room because your mother is waiting for you there."

When I saw the grief in my mother's face, tears flooded my eyes. I asked her, "How could this happen? I can't believe it! I just saw him this morning and he seemed so healthy!"

My mother said quietly, "He did not appear normal this morning; he told me that he had a severe headache. I had never seen him in such agony in all the time we've been married. He said he could not tolerate the severe pain. Usually he never complains, even when he is in severe pain. But this morning his complaining was so different, it seemed that he could not handle the pain and he took strong medication for his headache. I asked him to stay home and rest."

However, like all Japanese men, he would not listen to my mother. The more my mother pleaded with him, the angrier my

Do No Harm

father became. He told her, "I am a doctor. I know my body and the state of my health better than you do. Today I must perform an important procedure on an esophagus cancer patient that no one else can do except me. Don't worry about me. Once the medication works, I will be fine!"

Again, my mother said to him, "Maybe I don't know medicine because I am not a doctor. However, I am your wife and I know when something is wrong.

"Please don't go to the hospital today. Please! Today you look so pale and I have a feeling that your blood pressure is very high. You need to give yourself a rest. You can postpone the operation until tomorrow!"

But my father refused my mother's advice. "I will go to the hospital right now. My patient is waiting for me."

My mother held me close and the tears ran down her face as she remembered how once more she asked my father, "Please don't go to the hospital!"

She grasped my father's hand and pleaded with him. But he was determined and nothing was going to stop him.

Three days later, my father died. He never regained consciousness. My mother was only 38 years old. My mother knew that my father died so young because he literally worked himself to death.

The day my father died my mother said to me, "Taka! Please listen to me!

Someday you will follow in your father's footsteps and you also will be a doctor."

"I will love your father forever. Even though he is no longer alive, I will always be his wife. It is true that he was a good husband for me. He was a good doctor and a good man, but he was driven by his desire to compete with his father's accomplishments. Your father wanted to establish his personal fame and he was determined that he would be more successful and famous than his father."

"Since your grandfather established the Ohno Hospital over 30 years ago, many young doctors have come from all over

Japan in order to learn special operation techniques. Even though the salaries for them were low, they worked at the Ohno Hospital in order to learn. Because of the low salaries paid to the doctors, your grandfather accumulated a great sum of money to establish a new hospital. Your father was determined that your grandfather would not outdo him. Therefore, he was obsessed with building a bigger hospital for himself in Osaka."

"He worked everyday to establish this new hospital so that he would not be overshadowed by his father's accomplishments. He also struggled with the hospital union. When he became the director of the hospital, after his father retired, the hospital union became stronger. He has fought against the union and he started to drink to escape the pressure.

"Three days ago, he drank so much that he vomited in the taxi. The taxi driver was so angry because of the bad smell. I remember that he also had a very bad headache and he felt very ill that day. I am sure that it was his ambition to outdo his father and the struggle with the hospital union that ended up killing him. Even though he was a good doctor and a good man, he could never be satisfied with himself. He had become obsessed to conquer his personal demons and it was his obsession that eventually killed him."

As my mother continued, she breathed very deeply and looked directly into my eyes. It was clear that she wanted to make a point to me so that I would become affected by her words.

"Taka, what I would like to say to you is that you should never be a 'money' doctor. If you allow yourself to become driven by your ego or by money, your life will be short. However, if you will be a 'humanitarian' doctor, your life will be so full of happiness! And the people that you help will be forever grateful."

"Everybody will respect you and you will gain credibility. Credibility is something that no one else can give you because you have to earn it yourself. And once you gain credibility, no one can ever take it away from you but yourself."

Do No Harm

"Taka! You should become a humanitarian doctor!" "If you become a humanitarian doctor, God will always bless you. Your patients will always bless you and be grateful to you! If you are not a humanitarian doctor you will have the same fate as your father. Even if you are fortunate and live longer than he did, your heart will carry the heavy burden of knowing that you are not caring for people in a compassionate way."

"You will recognize this and your heart will trouble you until you come to the realization that you must change. Only you will have the power to change."

During the time that followed, while I was taking care of my cancer patients, I always remembered what my mother had told me, *"Taka, you must be a humanitarian doctor, not a doctor obsessed with fame or money!"*

As I watched my patients suffer in agony from taking the anticancer drug, I was experiencing my own torment as well. I was so internally torn that it felt as though I was injecting the 'Devil's Drug' into myself. The struggle I went through was my coming to terms with what I felt was the right action to take that would ultimately put my patients' best interest first. I was beginning to become consumed with the memory of my mother's words to me after my father's death. The memory of that tragic period of my life started to overwhelm me and I began to move slowly towards another direction of focus for myself.

I was increasingly moving away from the mental trap that told me I was helpless as an intern and that I was obligated to follow the professor's instructions. I was beginning to gain a confidence that told me when I would do something that goes against the core of my belief system, then I am not moving in the right direction for myself or for others. I was beginning to realize that I was not a humanitarian doctor. I had many personal struggles that I was trying to work through, and there were times I prayed for the physical and emotional strength to carry me through. I never wanted to become too busy or too preoccupied to lose the perspective of my wish to become a caring doctor.

Yoshitaka Ohno, M.D., Ph.D.

When my father died, I was just 16 years old, my brother was 17, and my sister was 15. Our mother wanted us all to become doctors. For two generations, the Ohno Hospital had been our family's business. As soon as I graduated medical school, my mother appointed me director of the Ohno Hospital. This was a tremendous burden upon me because I had never been trained in business management! I knew I was not yet prepared to be a doctor, let alone the director of a hospital.

My mother said, "I know you don't feel prepared to take the responsibility, Taka, but you must understand the importance of this situation!

"The present director at the Ohno Hospital is not part of the Ohno family. He is an outsider and he cannot possibly run the hospital in the family's best interest. I need you to run our hospital because you are the only family member right now who is in the position to handle this responsibility!"

"I understand that you have just graduated from medical school and that you need to do your internship at University Hospital. But you also need to devote time to Ohno Hospital as well. You have a commitment to insure that our hospital remains within the family.

"Taka, I insist that you to report to the Ohno Hospital immediately and fulfill your family duty as the hospital director!"

I was overwhelmed with what my mother had told me, "My brother is older than me, why can't he be the director of the Ohno Hospital?"

"Your brother won't be finished with his training from the Tokyo Women's University for another two or three years. When he is finished with his training he will return to Osaka and he will take over as the director. So until he finishes with his training, you will act as director. I know I am requiring a lot from you, but I have much faith that you will be able to handle the responsibility."

At the age of 25, my days were split between working at Ohno Hospital every day from early in the morning until 1:00

Do No Harm

PM. As hospital director, I was only a figurehead. I felt like an ornament inside a show window. I struggled every day. Every day was painful for me. I felt my rightful place was with my patients and that, of course, is where I desired to be. In the afternoon I would go over to the University Hospital to see my patients. My world seemed so crowded. In the morning I was the director of one hospital and in the afternoon I was a mere intern in training, learning how to take care of my patients! I set my daily schedule to concentrate my time on them. The meaning they brought to my life helped me get through the taxing responsibilities at Ohno Hospital.

Three nights a week I worked the midnight shift in the emergency ward at Ohno Hospital as well. I prayed to God many times to give me the strength and energy to continue with my day-to-day obligations. I prayed to God many times to give me insight and knowledge on how I could discover a more effective way to help my patients. One night, when I was unable to sleep, the memory of my paternal grandmother's experience with cancer brought me a new insight into my dilemma.

This very sad story occurred in 1968 while I was still a student at Kurume Medical School in Kyushu, Japan. I went home to Osaka, to visit my grandmother who was very ill and in the hospital. Because I was a medical student, and because no one was taking care of her properly, she begged me to help her.

"Taka, you are a medical student, so I know you definitely can help to stop my pain!

"I cannot tolerate this pain! Please ask the nurse to come and give me an injection that will stop my pain! Please hurry!"

My grandmother was suffering from colon cancer. About a year earlier she had noticed an abnormal feeling in her abdomen. She ignored the symptoms because she was afraid of the diagnosis. Her husband was Ryozo Ohno, my grandfather. He was a very famous surgeon who specialized in gastric cancer in Japan. Many times my grandmother had listened to the stories about this terrible cancer from my grandfather. She was afraid that she had this cancer and she did not want to go for a check-up. However, she began to suffer from diarrhea and constipation, and finally she developed blood in her stool. Sadly, when she finally went to the hospital for an examination, it was too late. Her colon cancer had already metastasized to other organs. She had an operation to remove the cancer, but not all of it could be taken out of her body. Her symptoms worsened day by day after the operation.

When I came home to Osaka and visited her in the hospital, I was shocked to see her appearance. I would never have recognized her. She looked like a completely different person. Her face was very brown from jaundice, due to liver deficiency, and she had lost over 50 pounds. Her eyes were yellow and her eyeballs protruded from their sockets. She looked like a living ghost.

My grandmother grasped my hand and begged me to give her a drug that would ease her pain. I was just a medical student so I could not administer drugs to her.

Due to over administration of the anticancer drug and other pain relievers, her skin had completely broken down. Her immune system had deteriorated as well. Medication would no longer work for her. When she drank water, she instantly would vomit. Due to not having control of her bowels and bladder, her room was filled with a foul smell and it was difficult to stay there for more than a few minutes at a time. Because of the foul smell, the nurses did not visit her room as often as they should have.

She was in a very sad and hopeless situation. I felt hopeless because I was so limited in what I could do to help her. She would scream to me again and again, "Taka help me! Help me!"

"O.K grandmother! I will try to help you! I will try to do what I can!"

But there was nothing I could do for her. The only thing I could do was hold her hand and give comfort to her. Or I would go to the nurse's station and ask them to help her, but they did not respond quickly because they were busy. They also didn't like to go into her room because of the terrible smell.

Do No Harm

The more I witnessed my grandmother living through this agony, the more I would ask myself, *"Why is it that modern medicine cannot do anything to help a patient in such agony?"*

Three days after I arrived to visit her, my grandmother died. She was 75 years old. After she died, I again seriously questioned my decision to become a doctor. I had felt so helpless trying to assist her. I was able to do nothing for her. Even though I was a medical student, all I was able to do was to go to the nurse's station and wait for a nurse to come into the room to help her. I loved my grandmother very much, yet I was inadequate when it came time to relieve her of her pain and discomfort. I struggled to determine if I really wanted to become a doctor.

After my grandmother's funeral and before I returned to medical school, I talked to my mother about my feelings.

"Mother, I want to quit medical school. I sincerely question whether I will make a good doctor."

My mother emphatically told me, "I know you feel discouraged, Taka, but there was nothing you could have done for your grandmother.

"You should continue with medical school and become a wonderful doctor. Your grandmother wanted you to finish medical school. She knew you would become a humanitarian doctor. She always told me that Yoshitaka should be like Dr. Albert Schweitzer, who went to Africa to take care of the native Africans and cured many of their diseases.

"Your grandmother had so much faith in you, so you need to stay in medical school. Then you can continue with your journey to become a truly humanitarian doctor who will help so many people."

Remembering what my grandmother had experienced in the end stages of her cancer, I realized that most cancer patients were not really being helped; and the side effects from their treatments made their cancer even more unbearable. I also realized that modern medicine really had not improved very much, from 1968 when my grandmother died. I decided that I needed to find a way to change the way cancer patients are treated so they have a better chance of survival.

I decided that I didn't want my father's premature death and my grandmother's suffering to be for nothing. I had lived through these tragic experiences for a reason and I knew that it was up to me to learn from these struggles. I knew that I had to find something new to help my patients. I was determined to discover a new way to solve the mystery of cancer.

The pathology department of Nara Medical University was well known for research. My father-in-law, Professor Tsubura, was the director of this department. My interest in research intensified, as I became more committed to discovering an alternative method of treatment for my patients.

Against my father-in-law's advice, I convinced him to allow me to do research in his department. My schedule certainly was overloaded, juggling my time between Ohno Hospital as director, and my internship at University Hospital. But I was determined to pursue research. So once a week I traveled to Nara, which was about an hour's drive from Osaka. There I would devote a morning to research. My interest in research grew as I realized that as I searched for answers to a cure for cancer, I was beginning to feel as though I had discovered something new for myself: Hope. It was the feeling of hope that I wanted so desperately to give to my patients.

I was determined that I would become a humanitarian doctor and nothing was going to stop me.

It takes courage to live in your truth.
It requires truth to be able to live courageously.

Chapter Three

The Maruyama Vaccine

*Once you step into the light you can stand still in it,
but you can never leave.
You will never be able to deny awareness.
Responsibility of right action will always remain within you.*

From the time I started medical school, I was aware of the Maruyama vaccine.

The Maruyama vaccine was named after Dr. Chisato Maruyama, a Japanese doctor who discovered it. I was familiar with this vaccine because it was a very controversial drug with the JFDA, even though it had been proven to cure cancer.

Dr. Chisato Maruyama, who died in 1995, had been a former honorary professor of dermatology at the Japan Medical University. According to Dr. Maruyama's book: ***Maruyama Vaccine Since Then***, every year the number of cancer patients increase by more than 60,000. In 1970 the estimated number of cancer patients was 120,000, but in 1980 that number increased to 160,000. In 1984 the number rose to 180,000 cancer patients.

In Japan, doctors use mostly chemotherapy for cancer patients. But the side effects, which include fever, vomiting, loss of appetite, hair loss and a decrease in blood count, are so strong that many cancer patients actually die from the side effects and not from the cancer. The Maruyama vaccine does not have any side effects for the cancer patient. The chemotherapy treatment kills all cells; it does not know how to differentiate between normal and cancerous cells, so it kills all of the cells that it comes into contact with. The Maruyama vaccine does not kill the cells; rather it increases the immune system function, helping kill the cancer cells without the horrors of strong side effects.

Yoshitaka Ohno, M.D., Ph.D.

Dr. Maruyama, a dermatologist, did research in skin tuberculosis. In 1944 he started to study a vaccine, which was derived from tuberculin bacteria in tuberculosis patients. Dr. Robert Koch was the first to discover the tuberculin treatment for tuberculosis patients in 1890, but the results were not beneficial. The side effects of fever and fatigue were too strong. Due to the side effects, the tuberculin vaccine lost credibility.

Dr. Maruyama felt that there was a poison in the tuberculin that caused the side effects. He knew that if the poison could be eliminated from the tuberculin, then he could use it successfully on his tuberculosis patients. He also knew that protein would cause the side effects, so he eliminated the protein from the tuberculin vaccine. This particular vaccine without the protein is known today as the Maruyama vaccine. He established the vaccination in 1952. He used it first on leprosy patients and discovered dramatic, positive results. Next, he used it on his skin tuberculosis patients with the same positive results.

One day in 1956, at the Japan Medical University, he came across the realization that leprosy patients who were given the tuberculin vaccine did not contract cancer. He conducted a study on his theory, which confirmed that this was valid. He decided first to use the Maruyama vaccination on an animal that had cancer, but the experiment failed. The difference of the antibodies between animals and humans is great. However, even though the animal experiment was not successful, he recognized there was a definite difference in the antibody make-up, so he proceeded to use the vaccination on a human being with cancer. In 1965, Dr. Maruyama tried the vaccine for the first time on a patient with end stage pancreatic cancer. She was a 52-year-old patient who was given two months to live. Dr. Maruyama administered the vaccination on his patient twice a week. Amazingly, after five months, her cancer had diminished! After nine months, her cancer was in a state of complete remission. Today, 35 years later, this cancer patient is alive and well, and still actively working in the same place of employment.

Do No Harm

In 1976, and after years of receiving dramatic results with his vaccination, Dr. Maruyama applied to the JFDA (Japan's FDA) with clinical data for the acceptance of his drug. In most cases, it takes the JFDA approximately one to two years to approve a new drug. However, it was evident that after several years, the JFDA was not going to approve the Maruyama vaccination. The JFDA determined that the data Dr. Maruyama had was false. Dr. Maruyama conducted several more successful experiments and provided clinical data again to the JFDA. Every time he was turned down. The reasons for denial were strictly political in nature and actually had nothing to do with the clinical data supporting the Maruyama vaccination. Around the same time that Dr. Maruyama had applied to the JFDA another doctor, a cancer specialist, also applied for approval with a similar drug, and was approved.

Japanese medical society looked down upon Dr. Maruyama because he was not a graduate from a prestigious school like the Tokyo University. There are over 100 medical universities in Japan, but only three are considered elite, or Ivy League status. Graduates from these universities are ranked high and given special privileges, which helps qualify them for prestigious awards like the Nobel Prize. Dr. Maruyama graduated from a less prestigious school, the Japan Medical University. If he were to win a Nobel Prize through the discovery, it would be an insult to the Japan Medical Society, especially the Tokyo University.

The three main universities in Japan control the JFDA and the pharmaceutical companies because of their influence. When a high staff member of the JFDA, who was a graduate of Tokyo University, asked the President of the Japan Medical University to have Dr. Maruyama fired, pressure was applied. If Dr. Maruyama were to gain fame because of his vaccine, it would be an embarrassment to the prestigious Japanese medical schools. Although Dr. Maruyama was not fired from his position, he was indeed isolated. He did not receive any support from his peers at the University and was ostrasized socially.

Yoshitaka Ohno, M.D., Ph.D.

Dr. Maruyama was a man of high principles. He would not accept money from the pharmaceutical companies like most of the doctors did. In Japan many doctors receive money from pharmaceutical companies to test new drugs. But, too often, the doctors do not apply the money to research. Dr. Maruyama was a humanitarian, much like Albert Schweitzer. Dr. Schweitzer was a Nobel Prize winner. Both men had the same vibration of spiritual energy. A challenged spirit goes out on a limb, putting the greater good of mankind first. It is these special people who ultimately make a profound difference in the world.

I decided I would secretly use the Maruyama vaccine on my patients. But I was aware that in order to help my patients by giving them the vaccination, I would have to enlist the help of their family members.

I called together the families of my breast cancer and bone tumor patients. This was a confidential meeting. I secretly arranged to have the meeting in the private room of one of my patients. After they had gathered together, I told them, "You should go to the Japan Medical University in Tokyo and obtain the Maruyama vaccine. This needs to be done immediately!

"Your only hope to save your loved one is this vaccination which has proven results of shrinking cancer cells.

"I cannot tolerate the continued use of the anticancer drug which I feel is the 'Devil's Drug'. This anticancer drug is not working on them and you are my only hope to go and get this drug!

"You should not waste any time so that I can start the new therapy right away!"

The families were so excited! They were willing to do whatever they could for their loved one. After we talked, I became very serious as I explained to them,

"Before you go to the Japan Medical University, I have to tell you that this must remain confidential. No one can talk about what I am doing, because if the hospital professor knew I was giving the Maruyama vaccination to my patients, I would lose my job.

Do No Harm

"You must not tell what we are doing to anyone. You have to promise that we will keep this a secret between us."

All of the family members nodded their heads and said, "Oh, yes! We promise!"

One of the family members said to me, "You are a hero to the patients who need this vaccination! Thank you. Thank you!"

I told them, "Thank you for the faith you have in me. Thank you very much!"

For the first time, I began to see hope in the faces of people. Every day they stood by while their loved ones suffered from anticancer drugs. Even though what I asked them to do was risky business, they were delighted to know that there was an alternative medication. I will never forget how good I felt that day just knowing that for once we all had a sense of hope.

Every day, the patients' charts were routinely monitored by the hospital supervisor and other medical staff members. Verification that all medications were given in a timely manner was constantly being documented. I had to figure out a way to get around the check-and-balance system that was making sure I was fulfilling my obligations.

After the family members obtained the Maruyama vaccine, I immediately proceeded to give the new medication to my patients. Twice a week when I had to administer the anticancer drug, I went to the nurse's station and requested the normal drug that was routinely given to the cancer patients. Under general procedure, a nurse would accompany me to the patient's room while I administered the vaccination. However, I told the nurses that I would not need their assistance and I proceeded to my patient's room, trying not to draw attention to myself.

Tucked in a pocket inside of my hospital coat was a vial of the Maruyama vaccine. I flushed the anticancer drug down the toilet in my patient's bathroom and quickly injected the Maruyama vaccination into them instead. I then falsified the hospital records to show I had given the patient the anticancer drug. I proceeded upon this secret mission twice a week for both

Yoshitaka Ohno, M.D., Ph.D.

of my patients. As uncomfortable as I was about the 'dishonesty' of my action, I was not being tormented anymore by my heart. I knew I was doing what was the greater good for my patients and that awareness kept me in balance with my conscience.

One month after I started administering the Maruyama vaccine, amazing results occurred. After reviewing the X-rays from the breast cancer patient, I noticed a definite difference! Her cancer had started to shrink! I was elated! It was one of the most exciting moments in my life! At first I thought it was all my imagination, but after closer analysis of the X-rays, I determined that a miracle had taken place! Shortly thereafter, I began giving the vaccination to the young girl with the bone tumor and her tumor had started to shrink as well! The excitement was unbelievable! However, I had a dilemma because I could not share the results with any other doctors!

Two months later, both tumors were much smaller. The patients' conditions were definitely improving as they gained back their appetites, gained weight and started to generally feel much better.

After three months, X-rays showed that their tumors had nearly disappeared. I was now seriously considering discharging the patients from the hospital! They were coming alive again, and their family members were thrilled to watch as their health improved daily!

But before I was able to discharge my patients, something terrible happened. The professor was made aware that I had been using the Maruyama vaccine on these cancer patients. He was furious with me and immediately called me into his office.

"What did you do to my patients? They are so important to me because I need to see if my new drug is working or not! You have destroyed my research because you decided to use the Maruyama vaccine on them!

"How could you do such a stupid thing? Do you know how many times I have given instructions not to use the Maruyama vaccine?

Do No Harm

"Even though you are well known and well liked, you have used this worthless vaccination on my patients. You know the rules that if you disobey my orders, you will be immediately fired!"

I tried to explain to him, "Whatever rule or unwritten law, if the anticancer drug is tormenting the patients and they are not getting better, we should stop using the drug right away and decide to do what is in the best interest of the patient!"

The professor listened to what I had to say and shouted back at me with anger,

"Get out of here! You are fired! Leave right now! I never want to see your face again!"

After I left the professor's office another doctor said to me, "Are you crazy?" Why didn't you obey the professor's instructions? Even though his instructions may be wrong, we must always obey him!

"Even if the professor says, 'This is not cancer' and we know it is cancer, we still must agree that it is not cancer!

"However, you did not obey his instructions and it is too late for you now. Did you stop to think about what you have done to yourself?

"You will never get another job again in the medical field because the professor will create obstacles for you! You were very foolish!"

All the interns and doctors blamed me. However, I have never regretted that I lost my job over doing what I knew was right for my patients. Even in that moment, I was proud of myself. I stood up for what I believed in and I stood up for what I believed was best for my patients.

My desk was cleared out that very same day. The only regret I ever felt was that I would never see my patients again, and I was concerned what would happen to them after I had left.

I went to my patient's room to say goodbye before I left the hospital. She asked me, "Why are you leaving this hospital? You have done nothing wrong! You are a humanitarian doctor and you have helped us!

Yoshitaka Ohno, M.D., Ph.D.

"If you did something bad, we could understand, but you have helped us get better! If you had done something wrong that hurt us, we would understand why you have been fired, but our health has improved!"

Even though I could not answer my patient's questions, I took to heart what she was saying to me.

Then I said to her, "Whatever the reasons, I have been fired. I wish to thank you all very much for your support. I hope you will continue to get healthy and be discharged from the hospital soon. I thank you all for supporting me."

Just as I turned to leave the room, a voice cried out to me. It was my breast cancer patient.

"Please, Dr. Ohno! Please don't leave me! If you leave, I will also leave this hospital! I will follow you to another hospital!"

She was crying and sobbing. She jumped into my arms and continued to sob.

The other patients in the room started to cry and one of them said, "You are our only hope!"

When I heard these words, I started to cry. I could not stop crying. My breast cancer patient hugged me and said, "Please don't leave us! You are our only hope! You can't leave us now because we need you!"

I was appreciative that they wanted me to stay. I said to them, "I was very happy to have been your doctor. Thank you very much for your appreciation!"

"I hope and pray that you will be discharged very soon from the hospital and that I will see you one day again!"

"My dream is to be a good doctor, a humanitarian doctor, and you gave me the opportunity to learn to be one! I'll never forget you!

I left my heart in that hospital room that day. My heart was breaking, as I had to leave my patients behind in a state of tears and fear and confusion. I was especially sad as I turned around one more time before I left the hospital ward and saw my breast

Do No Harm

cancer patient being held and comforted by the other patients. I attempted to fight back tears as I left the room for the last time.

There had been many times during those three months that I had wondered how this would end. I knew that eventually someone would discover what I had been doing. But because the vaccination was successful in both of my patients, I was hoping that once the discovery was made, everything would be all right. My wishful thinking had been too optimistic. I prayed for myself. I prayed for my patients.

Yoshitaka Ohno, M.D., Ph.D.

Hokkaido, Japan

Healing my heart and taking a break.

Just after I was fired, I decided to get away from Osaka and take a much-needed break. I went to Hokkaido, which is in the north of Japan. There are many hot springs there and it is a very beautiful and peaceful area. I love hot springs and thought that this would be the perfect place for me to go to attempt to heal my heart and work through the stress of running the hospital.

After I arrived at the hotel, I went to a hot spring spa. After nearly an hour of bathing and relaxing, I decided to do some window shopping at a souvenir shop in the hotel. I noticed a young boy playing at the game machine. He was about 15 years of age. Usually I would not have paid any attention to a boy playing the popular game, but this boy had a bandage wrapped around his head and his face was very pale in color. It was obvious that he had very little energy and he wasn't enjoying the game. He seemed to be very sick.

I decided to go over and play the game with him. During the game, I noticed that he must have had some kind of operation. I didn't want to ask him because that was his private business. Thirty minutes later a lady came over to us and said.

"Thank you very much for playing with my son! I haven't seen him smile and enjoy himself since he had his operation! Thank you very much!"

I told her, "It has been my pleasure, I am Dr. Ohno."

When the mother realized I was a doctor, she explained her son's story. "My son is suffering from a malignant brain tumor that he's had for about a year.

First, he had complained of having headaches and I ignored him because I thought he was trying to stay home from school. But his headaches became so severe that I knew I had to bring him to the hospital for examination. The doctor did a MRI and

Do No Harm

discovered the brain tumor. A biopsy was done to check the tumor and we found out that it was malignant.

"The doctor did an operation but the tumor had already metastasized and spread to his brain. The tumor could not be removed, so the doctor decided to start radiation therapy instead.

"One month ago, X rays at the hospital were taken and the doctor explained to us that the tumor had actually grown and was larger than it was a month ago before we started the radiation therapy."

"Unfortunately, there is nothing we can do for your son. The only thing you can do now is return home and let him live out the rest of his life there."

The mother was starting to cry as she recalled asking the doctor, "What! I can't understand what you have just told me, because before you said that the radiation therapy was the best treatment!

"Can't we continue to give him the radiation therapy to keep the growth rate down?"

But the doctor said, "We have done everything we could but the therapy is just not working. It is not stopping his cancer from growing and spreading."

Fighting back the tears, the mother said she had asked the doctor, "Tell me honestly, how long does my son have to live?"

"Your son has about three months to live."

"I couldn't believe that they gave him only three months to live! He is only 15 years old! His life is just beginning!

"I asked them if there was another therapy they could try. Then I asked the doctor, if his son was faced with the same situation, wouldn't he want to make sure he was doing everything he possibly could to save his son's life?

"But the doctor could not answer me. He only said that he was sorry. He said,

There is nothing else we can do for your son. All we can suggest to you is that whatever your son wants you to do, you should do for him. Just make him comfortable and try to keep him happy.

Yoshitaka Ohno, M.D., Ph.D.

The mother was crying as she finished her story. Then she asked me, "Why is God punishing my son? Did he do something to God, something bad? I have never done anything bad and my ancestors have not done anything bad! I don't understand why my son is going through this punishment. We are all so miserable. I wish God would decide to punish me and not my son!"

We stood there in silence for a long time. I had no idea what I could say to the boy's mother to give her comfort. While we were talking, the boy had continued to play the video game.

I stood there thinking that there had to be a reason for me to meet the boy and his mother. I had just come to Hokkaido to heal myself from the painful experience of trying to help my cancer patients. And here I was, once again, being brought face to face with yet another situation of someone that was fighting for his life. I tried to think of what I could do for the boy and his mother.

Finally, the boy's mother broke the silence and said, "I know my son only has three months to live and that he will not survive. But there are many cancer patients who continue to suffer. Please, Dr. Ohno, try to find a new therapy for cancer, one that doesn't destroy the body like radiation or chemo. Please find a new cure for people like my son!"

I told her, "I will do my best. I don't know exactly what I can do, but I will try to do my best."

After returning to Osaka from Hokkaido, I told my mother about the incident with the young cancer patient and his mother. My mother said to me, "You have had a good experience, Taka.

"If you had not gone to Hokkaido, you would never have had such an experience. You should try to find a way to answer the boy's mother's request. You see, every patient is anxiously waiting for good news. Everywhere you go, people are looking for someone like you to help them. I believe nobody will be able to help these people but you. You should study more and search for new and creative ideas. Not a new anticancer drug that will be painful to the patient, but a true cure. This is your mission.

Do No Harm

Even though this is a very big challenge, no one can do this but you. God had given you this chance. You need to find an answer to help cancer patients!"

My mother continued, "In order for you to do your best job, you should go to Nara Medical University to do research full time in pathology. The pathology department is always searching for new ways to cure disease. You can concentrate on research and pursue your studies there."

After I talked to my mother, I discussed the idea with my father-in-law, Professor Tsubura. He agreed that it would be beneficial for me to join him in the pathology department. Before I went to Nara Medical University, I met an old friend of mine who was an intern at University Hospital, where I had recently been fired. "How are my patients," I asked. "Are they taking the anticancer drug?"

Then I heard the sad news. "Taka, I dread being the one to tell you your breast cancer patient is dead. But she did not die from the cancer. She committed suicide!"

"Suicide!" I screamed. I thought I had heard him incorrectly.

"Suicide!" he confirmed.

"How could she have done such a thing?"

"Since you left the hospital, she asked the nurses about you every day."

She continually asked, **"When is Dr. Ohno returning to the hospital? When will Dr. Ohno be back?"**

"The nurses were instructed to not answer any questions because the professor warned them not to talk about you."

Your breast cancer patient would say to me, *"I can't wait to see Dr. Ohno!"*

Why have you quit giving me the Maruyama vaccine?"

"She always asked the doctors to give her the Maruyama vaccine, but they continued giving her the tormenting anticancer drug. Since she could not tolerate the anticancer drug, she finally decided to commit suicide."

I was told that it happened on a very cold winter day. There was nobody on the twelfth floor of the hospital except for her.

Yoshitaka Ohno, M.D., Ph.D.

She arranged her shoes neatly and climbed up and over the window guard and jumped. When somebody discovered her body on the ground, her body was completely crushed from the impact of the fall. The ambulance was immediately called, but it was too late.

There was one thing she had left behind. On her bed was a letter for me.

To Dr. Ohno!

Thank you very much for your warm heart. I was so happy since I met you because you gave me the Maruyama vaccine. That worked so well for me. When I was on the anticancer drug, I was in a living nightmare because of the strong side effects. I always asked you to please help me die because I could not tolerate the strong side effects from this drug. You changed the anticancer drug to the Maruyama vaccination and I went from Hell to Heaven! After you started this vaccination, I definitely felt that I would be able to be discharged from the hospital and return to my home. However, when they found out that you were using the vaccination, they fired you.

After you were fired from the hospital, I just lay crying in my bed. "Why did Dr. Ohno leave?" I kept asking.

Even though I asked the nurse for your address they would not give it to me because of the hospital professor's orders. Then they started the anticancer drug again after they quit giving me the Maruyama vaccine. I asked them to please give me the Maruyama vaccination! But they never listened to my pleas and continued to give me the anticancer drug. Soon I started having the strong side effects again. I could not tolerate them. I finally decided to choose the easiest way to go to God. Please forgive me that I lost my spirit to fight for my life.

But I never forgot your warm heart; I will never forget your warm heart. Please give your warm heart to other cancer patients because they are waiting for you. They are waiting for you to help them. I hope you will continue to give hope to your patients. I am sure you can give them the hope because you are a completely different kind of doctor.

Good bye, Dr. Ohno! I am watching you from heaven!

When I read her suicide letter I couldn't stop crying. I felt guilty because if I were still at the hospital, she would never have done this. I had many unanswered questions in my mind but it was too late now for regret. I went to her funeral. Her face was beautiful, such a beautiful and peaceful face. To look at her peacefulness now, I would never have imagined that she had such a struggle and a fight with her cancer. I imagined that she was beside me and telling me, *"I am so glad to see you! I have missed you! Please take care of me again."* However, she would never say these words to me again.

A few days later I went back to visit her grave. I told her, "I will be a humanitarian doctor. I will do my best to find a new idea that will give hope to cancer patients. Please watch over me and bless me with your wonderful heart. Your loving heart will help to lead me to succeed and to discover a new idea that will fight disease."

After I made my promise at her grave, I committed myself to research in pathology. I worked very hard learning about the causes of cancer and how to stop it. I felt like I was a student again, studying very hard. I never experienced such intensity in my studies. It seemed like I was studying 24 hours a day! But whenever I felt tired and afraid that I would lose my fighting spirit to study, I would look at her picture and her smiling face to give me encouragement. I always felt she was watching over me while I did my research.

I would often talk to my mother for encouragement. I have appreciated so very much the unconditional love and support I have received from her all through my life. I know that my destiny is to help people heal and feel better. My goal is to find a way to stop the progression of diseases during aging.

Yoshitaka Ohno, M.D., Ph.D.

If it weren't for my family's history and my patients' tragedies, I would not understand the importance of being a humanitarian doctor. I believe that a powerful source of energy has been given to me, and a spiritual guide has been leading me in the direction of my destiny.

Dare to be what you are meant to be~ Do what you are meant to do~

And then Life will provide the means for you to do it and to be it.

Chapter Four

The Healing Process Continues At Nara Medical Hospital

As you grow in awareness you will simultaneously develop wisdom, release pain and learn to rise above aspects of your life that do not serve your greater purpose.

Two years after my mother appointed me to the position of medical director at Ohno Hospital, my brother, Yoshioki Ohno, returned home to Osaka. Yoshioki had completed his training from Tokyo Women's University, where he had learned several new surgical techniques that included a specialized procedure for breast cancer. Subsequently, Yoshioki took over the position of medical director of the hospital. This enabled me to move to Nara with my wife Akiko, where I went to work full time doing research in the pathology department at the Nara Medical Hospital.

Even though I had discovered a strong interest in research, the decision to go to the pathology department in Nara was difficult for me. In the Japanese culture, the family name is a place of honor. To honor and protect the family name is very important. Leaving the Ohno Hospital in Osaka as director was leaving a place that represented our family name and family honor. But I knew that I was meant to do research. I knew that all things in my life were for a reason. I remembered the days at University Hospital. Had the professor not used the tormenting anticancer drug on my patients, I would never have had to go to Nara Medical Hospital to do research. Then I wouldn't have discovered my interest and passion for research. I believed then, as I do now, that all of the events in my life have been an invisible force, guiding me and aiding me in the journey towards my destiny.

I enjoyed my research position at Nara Hospital. Professor Tsubura, my father-in-law, was a wonderful person to work for. Since I had lost my own father at such a young age, Professor Tsubura became a father figure to me. He was the perfect role model for me to learn from. He was kind and compassionate to everyone. He taught me the true meaning of humanitarianism. He believed so much in research because he truly wanted to find answers that would help people. I found a new purpose for my life, and I valued the opportunity to change the direction of my career.

The pathology department's research was directed towards finding a cure for breast cancer. At that time a discovery had been made, detecting the hereditary factor of breast cancer in mice. I had supposed that Professor Tsubura would instruct me to concentrate on pursuing this research, but he had other ideas for me. He encouraged me to begin a new research project that had not been done before, a research project on bacteria. This research was to be done to determine the relationship between bacteria and cancer. This was an opportunity that would prove to be very beneficial for my personal and professional growth, and would ultimately lead to my earning a Ph.D. There would be another twist in my working in cancer research. Cancer would enter into and have an effect upon my life once again. This time cancer would make its presence known in a way that was too close to home. This time cancer would threaten my mother's life.

1980
My mother discovers a breast tumor.

It was early in the morning and my mother was taking her bath. As she was drying herself, she noticed something abnormal in her breast. She pressed harder into the tender area

Do No Harm

and felt a tumor. She called my brother, Yoshioki, and asked him to come over to the house to examine her.

Yoshioki called me later that day. "Taka, I examined our mother this morning, and I have bad news! I think she has breast cancer!"

"What! Are you sure she has breast cancer? How can you be certain? You might be wrong with your diagnosis!"

"Taka, breast cancer is my specialty. I can tell by experience, when I touch a tumor, I can distinguish if it is malignant or benign.

"I believe her tumor is malignant!"

"Yoshioki, even though you are a specialist, you are not God! There is a possibility that you could be wrong! You are human and you may sometimes misdiagnose what you think is malignant!"

"Taka, listen to me...calm down and don't be so upset! Getting upset isn't going to help mother now!"

"But this is our mother," I protested. "Perhaps you are too close to the situation. Did you do a mammogram or ultrasound?"

"Not yet."

"Then until we have proof, you cannot be positive that she has breast cancer!"

"You are right, Taka, I have no clinical proof, but we do not have the luxury of time on our side.

After I run more tests and I am sure, Mother has asked me to perform the operation and I will fulfill her wishes. We will do surgery as soon as possible!"

Our mother was then 60 years old. After she called Yoshioki to examine her, she knew she wouldn't trust anyone else to perform her operation.

"Yoshioki, I want you to perform my operation. I will be so happy if you can do this for me. I don't want another doctor to do my operation. Please, promise me that you will take care of me!"

My brother took a deep breath and made his promise to her.

Yoshitaka Ohno, M.D., Ph.D.

Before the operation, a sample of her tumor was sent directly over to the pathology department at Nara Medical Hospital. I checked the sample myself to determine if it was malignant or benign.

My mother's tumor was malignant! I asked my father-in-law to re-check my diagnosis. I wanted to make sure that I wasn't reading the tests wrong. He verified my diagnosis and we immediately confirmed the malignancy to Yoshioki, who was at that moment preparing our mother for surgery. I looked at the cancer cells from my mother's body and I asked God:

"Why must you take my mother? Why can't you come and take me instead? I cannot stand the thought of my mother being tormented by the pain caused from cancer! Take me instead! Take me instead!"

I prayed for my mother. And I prayed for Yoshioki. Performing surgery on one's own mother was an exceptionally difficult task. I truly felt compassion for him, and I prayed to God to give him the strength and courage to perform this delicate operation.

Can we learn to finally awaken to the slumbering within ourselves and to hear the echoing of all our worries, fears and negative sounds?
And can we just see them crumbling and falling away into the nothingness from where they came from...

Ohno Hospital Operating Room

The door opened and Dr. Yoshioki Ohno quietly came in. Six of the surgical team were already prepared and waiting. He just stood behind the door and looked around with a keen eye. The green hospital garment he wore just fit him. The expression on his face was serious and centered. He looked as he normally

Do No Harm

did during any routine surgery. If he was feeling anxious or excited, he never allowed it to show.

Piercing through his surgical mask, his eyes were sharp and keen. You could sense that he brought into the room a strong spiritual energy. This energy transferred to everyone who was in the room. Anyone who had been apprehensive and tense before he entered into the room became affected by his calm and spiritual energy. He looked around the operating room and went directly over to the wall to look at mother's mammography. The room remained eerily quiet. After he reviewed the mammography, the surgeon assisting him said,

"Dr. Ohno, everything is ready."

Yoshioki looked down slightly and nodded his head. Even though his assistant was only 30 years old, he already had a reputation as a skilled doctor. Yoshioki was only 34 years old, but had already perfected his surgical skills, which were well known at the Tokyo Women's University.

The professor he studied under was a famous breast cancer surgeon who taught Yoshioki all of the newest techniques. He had mastered his training and although he was young, he had performed over 100 breast cancer operations. He had mastered the new techniques.

The Ohno Hospital has 500 beds. Even though they have many good surgeons there, Yoshioki is among the best. His name is rapidly becoming known in Japan.

Since Yoshioki had come to Ohno Hospital as medical director, everyone had been very impressed with his surgical skills. He was praised for his abilities and the reputation of Ohno Hospital continued to grow.

In the operating room, our mother lay sleeping. Yoshioki approached the table and looked down on her. Our mother had never remarried after our father's death. It was she who kept the family together and provided the leadership to the Ohno Hospital. Even though she had never worked before our father's death, she had helped to manage the hospital for almost 20 years after her marriage. She was a woman of conviction and courage.

Yoshitaka Ohno, M.D., Ph.D.

She was a mother who supported and helped her children. She was indeed a very special person whom everyone cared for.

The operating room was filled with doctors who were there to watch the new technique that Yoshioki was going to perform. Yoshioki looked to the anesthesiologist. The professor of the anesthesiology department requested that he personally wanted to handle the anesthesia for our mother's, surgery. The anesthesiologist looked at our mother and confirmed that the anesthetic had made her comfortable and ready.

Yoshioki took his position and checked everything such as surgical knives, respirator, anesthesia equipment, and so on. Once he was satisfied that everything was in order he said, "Let's start the operation."

The atmosphere was tense at first. Yoshioki's right hand reached out to the nurse.

The nurse passed him the surgical knife. The surgical knife met the skin at a 90-degree angle and cut through cleanly. Blood spattered. The assistant surgeon immediately stopped the bleeding. I could feel that Yoshioki and he were one in body and spirit.

Yoshioki was filled with confidence. "Electric knife." The nurse passed the electric knife. Everyone in the room seemed frozen.

I could sense that they were all thinking, *He's using an electric knife, not a scalpel?*

When an electric knife cuts into the subcutaneous tissue, it cuts cleaner, with less bleeding than a scalpel. However, the temperature of the blade becomes extremely hot. It takes a skilled surgeon to not burn the skin of the patient. This is the procedure that was to make Yoshioki famous in Japan.

Yoshioki found the tumor, which was the size of a walnut. He checked to see if it had metastasized to the lymph nodes. He did a liver scan and found no evidence of a tumor. He was relieved to find that the cancer had not spread. Yoshioki kept his emotions to himself even though he was very happy about the

Do No Harm

discovery. He had told himself at the beginning of the operation, "This is not my mother, this is my patient."

Before the surgery had begun, he decided to perform a radical mastectomy, which involves removal of the affected breast, along with the underlying pectoral muscles and axillary lymph nodes. This is because cancerous cells usually metastasize through the lymphatic system or the blood.

The surgery took two hours. In the waiting room, our whole family prayed for Yoshioki and our mother. Two hours seemed like twelve. Finally, the nurse came in and gave us the good news.

"The operation is over and your mother is fine. Dr. Yoshioki did an excellent job and everyone in the hospital is very proud of him!"

After the operation, I went looking for Yoshioki. I found him in the doctor's lounge next to the operating room. He was surrounded by the doctors who had been in attendance. They were congratulating him on his technique. When I saw him, he looked exhausted.

"Yoshioki, are you all right?" I asked.

"I am fine, Taka."

"Congratulations and thank you very much!" I said.

Yoshioki just nodded. I know the pressure he was under since the moment he decided to do the operation must have been constantly building inside of him. I had tremendous respect for him, not just as a doctor or as my brother, but as a person. He is truly one of the greatest doctors in the world. After I talked to him for a little while, I left him to rest.

As I walked out the door he said to me, "If someone were to ask me to do this again, I am not sure I would be able to do it. I never realized the degree of inner strength I would have to draw from in order to operate on our mother."

He never showed anyone how tired he was or the pressure he was under, because he was director of Ohno Hospital and had to keep up a strong appearance. My sister- in- law had later told me,

"I have never seen your brother so exhausted since we have been married. When he came back home he went straight to bed. It seemed as though he was sick from exhaustion and the pressure of your mother's operation."

I knew she was right. No son can do an operation on his mother and not be affected by the strain. I was proud of Yoshioki and I was equally thankful to God that everything had turned out positively.

Thirty minutes after the operation, my mother was transferred to a private room for recuperation. She was awake when I went in to see her.

"Mother, how are you. How do you feel?"

"I am fine."

"What do you feel knowing that Yoshioki performed your operation?"

She said, "I trusted him completely and I had no cause to worry."

I would never forget her words. I realized how extremely important trust between patient and doctor is. Trust is faith in action and without trust, fear sets in. When fear is present, the body's immune system does not function to full capacity. I believe there is a spiritual energy that transcends through both the doctor and the patient, which promotes a healing consciousness.

After my brother took my tissue samples of my mother's breast and lymph nodes, he brought them to me to take to the pathology department at Nara Medical Hospital. He wanted to double check if the cancer had not metastasized to the lymph nodes.

In the pathology department I called to Professor Tsubura, "Professor Tsubura, I am ready to prepare my mother's histological findings."

Professor Tsubura answered me "You should bring it over to me immediately. I will confirm whether or not the cancer has metastasized."

Do No Harm

I brought him the samples. One minute passed and he said nothing. Two minutes passed and he was still silently studying the samples. It seemed like an eternity.

After three minutes, he turned to me and said, "Congratulations, Dr. Ohno, I am very happy to tell you that your mother's cancer has not metastasized!"

"I am equally happy because you are my son-in-law and I would not have wanted to be the one to give you sad news if this was not the case! I am so happy! You can relax now. I believe your mother is going to be just fine!"

When I heard the good news from my father-in-law, I jumped up and down with joy. I immediately called my brother with the results. Yoshioki was not totally surprised because he had already confirmed that there was no metastasis to the lymph node. According to him, seeing and touching is believing, and he had not seen any indication of metastasis in our mother. But all the same, he was still relieved once again to hear the pathology results confirm what he already believed.

Three days after her operation, I visited my mother in the hospital room. I told her the good news that the cancer had not metastasized. She was very happy and said to me,

"I am not surprised by your good news. I am the happiest lady in the world right now! I am so thankful! No one could have such an experience, to have a son perform an operation on his mother! Even though there are two to three billion people in this world, think of the chances of this happening!"

"Taka, I want to tell you that I am so fortunate to have Yoshioki as such a wonderful son who had the strength to operate on his mother! I felt Yoshioki's strength, and it reminded me so much of your father."

"But I need to tell you something very important that happened to me, just as I was beginning to fall asleep under the anesthesia. I saw your father come to me. He was very loving and concerned, and he said these words to me,"I am very appreciative that my son Yoshioki can do this operation for you. Even though I could not reach my goal of watching the Ohno

Hospital grow, my son Yoshioki will carry on for me. I am very happy and at peace. And I appreciate all that you have done. Even though I died and left you at such a young age with our three children to raise, you did such an excellent job all by yourself. Please don't worry about this operation. I know you will be fine."

"Yoshiko, I will always watch over you and our children."

My mother had tears in her eyes as she shared this dream with me. She went on and explained to me, "Taka, even though I lived through such a tragedy at a young age, I always would tell myself, 'Don't give up!' I could not allow myself to give up because I had three wonderful children to raise. I was focused on doing the best I could to be the best mother I could be. I am so proud of Yoshioki that he has become such a wonderful surgeon, and I am so proud of you, Taka, because you are turning into such a good doctor."

She continued. "I went to a fortune teller once when I was young and she told me,

> *Your young life will be very sad and terrible. But your old age will become very happy. You should be patient and never give up because you have a bright future.*

"Taka, I remember her words and I feel she was right. I have a very fortunate life and I have much happiness ahead of me."

It was good to see my mother in such good spirits. We talked for awhile more and then I got up to leave so she could get some rest. I was almost out of the room when she called me back, "Taka!"

"I nearly forgot to tell you! While I was under the anesthesia, I had a wonderful dream about you! I dreamed that you won the Nobel Prize about something you did with water!" I know it was you, not Yoshioki. I don't know why I had this dream, but I somehow believe it is true!"

Do No Harm

When I heard her dream, I started to cry. I was crying because of the unyielding faith she had in me. She had a great deal of trust in what she knew I could accomplish. But when I heard her story about the water, it was difficult for me to understand how I would win the Nobel Prize because of water. Instead of water, I felt that my research in the field of bacteria and its relationship with cancer was how I would earn my recognition in the future.

After my mother suffered from her experience with breast cancer, I focused on the research project that my father-in-law, Professor Tsubura, assigned to me. This research would determine the correlation between breast cancer and bacteria. It seemed from the onset that it would be very difficult to establish evidence on this relationship, but I had a strong feeling that I could do it. This research would take four years to complete.

I discovered that bacteria are not the enemy we have always believed. According to the results of my experiments, I discovered that if we destroy the bacteria in our body, we would die because bacteria are necessary to help keep our bodies stable. The presence of bacteria in our body is necessary to immune system functioning. If there were no bacteria in our bodies, we would lose our ability to fight off invasion of toxins and pathogens, and we would die. This was the subject of my thesis, which was published in The Journal of Nara Medical Association. Because of my findings, Professor Tsubura was credited for the outstanding research of the Nara pathology department. As a result of this study, I was awarded my Ph.D.

Although I was very happy to have accomplished what I had set out to do, there were decisions that I needed to make about my future. Most doctors, after receiving their Ph.D., normally continue with clinical studies. Remaining in pathology would not offer the same income potential as a medicinal practice. But I did not want to get involved with a clinical practice. There were always the sales agents of drug companies who were always waiting to see me. I was not interested in wasting my time talking about the new drugs they were promoting. If I do not believe in a drug and feel it is not for the best interest of the patient, I will not be bothered. And I certainly was not going to get caught up in accepting money or other bribes from the drug salesmen.

After awhile, I became tired from the constant stream of salesmen and their valueless drugs. I knew I had to figure out which direction I was going to take and I knew my mother could help in rendering me with some advice. About three weeks before I received my Ph.D., I came back to Osaka from Nara to visit my mother and discuss my plans with her.

"Taka, what do you know? What is it you want to accomplish?", my mother asked.

I told her how I felt about clinical practice and I truly did not want to go in that direction.

"Mother, I cannot tolerate the constant pressure from the drug companies. Too many hospitals deal with this issue. I also feel that I don't want to stay in the pathology department in Nara, because I am the son-in-law of the professor. There are researchers there who are jealous of me because Professor Tsubura has given me special opportunities and they resent me for that. I am thankful to him, but I want to venture out and create my own career in medicine."

"I am really struggling with this decision. I am here to ask you what you think I should do. I have always valued your opinion and I will consider what you say very carefully."

"Taka, I agree with you that you should not go back to practicing medicine at a hospital. I also agree that it is not in you"

"I have thought for some time now that you may have a much better opportunity in a foreign country. This will give you the opportunity to grow, and help you to find your true calling, your destiny.

"If you remain in Japan, you will always be under the influence of the Ohno family name. You need to become your own man without the strong influence and power of the Ohno

Do No Harm

family. It is the family name, which has always been a protection for you.

" Taka, who will protect you after I die? Nobody will protect you except yourself. As long as you stay in Japan you will never find out who you are because you will constantly be in the shadow of the Ohno family.

"I feel that if you stay in Japan you will become defeated because there are so many unscrupulous people in the medical field here. If you stay in Japan, you will eventually lose your humanitarian ideals, because the challenges will be too difficult for you to continuously rise above them. Since I had the experience of being married to your father, I know how greedy the Japanese Medical Society can be.

"Too many people who know our family are always trying to become friends with us. But they are liars who really just want our money.

"I don't want you to be part of our medical society, Taka. I want you to grow into a good, humanitarian doctor. The Japanese medical society will not allow you the opportunity to achieve this.

"Taka, you are going to have to leave Japan."

Mother took a sip of her tea. Even though she believed in what she was telling me, I could see that it was difficult for her. I knew that she was trying to do what she felt was best for me and I appreciated her devotion.

"Taka, I have a story to tell you. I want to tell you what your father's mother, your grandmother, Mikino, told me before she died. She had called for me right before she passed away. I will always remember her words. These were the words from her deathbed:

"Yoshiko! She said, I apologize to you. I am on my knees to you and I want to beg your pardon. Since you married my son, Yoshio, you have done an excellent job as a wife for him and as a daughter- in- law for me.

From early in the morning until midnight you have worked very hard every day. I never expected you to do such a fine job.

Yoshitaka Ohno, M.D., Ph.D.

I always gave you so much work to do. I thought you would go back to your home in Tokyo if I forced too much work upon you. I remember you waking up at 5:00 A.M. to take care of the chickens and the rest of the farm. After you finished that job, you would prepare our food and then you took care of the family business the rest of the day. After Yoshio died, I was sure you would return to Tokyo.

"But you never complained, even though the work was so hard. You even went to work at the Ohno Hospital to help manage the hospital employees. Many nights you would return home after 7:00 P.M. and still take care of your three young children. You taught your children how to write good Japanese characters through your devotion and your commitment to them. Many nights you did not go to bed until after midnight.

You continued to work very hard for 20 years after Yoshio died. You took care of me and Ryouzo, your father-in-law, even you had surgery. Our own two daughters do not take care of us the way you do.

"Yoshiko, I appreciate you for all you have given to our family. You have given the Ohno family two sons. I was only able to have one son. I love both Yoshioki and Yoshitaka very much. And it is so important that they will continue the Ohno family blood line."

"I hope that Yoshioki will become the president of the Ohno family business someday. But I fear that if Yoshitaka becomes the assistant president, they will not have a good relationship. I fear that this will divide our family. This will bring shame to the family name."

"I think it would be better if Yoshitaka will move away to Hawaii or the mainland of America. Yoshitaka has a strong character that can be used for the good of humanity. Even though he will be presented with many challenges from living in a foreign country, he will conquer those difficulties and realize his destiny."

"I hope that when the day comes, Yoshiko, that you will tell Yoshitaka my dreams for him."

Do No Harm

"Taka, I understand your grandmother's words better now and I agree with what she told me. I believe as she did that you should go to America and work at becoming a humanitarian doctor. Your brother was destined to take care of the Ohno Hospital and I can continue to help him there. I do not want you to worry about us. I want you to go to America and do what will make you happy."

"Where in America should I go?" I asked.

"We should ask Professor Tsubura for his advice."

"Mother, I know that he will feel that I should go to the Ohno Hospital and he will be very surprised to hear that I am considering moving to America. But I know that he will be able to recommend a good place for me so that I can pursue my study and further my career in research."

After I received my Ph.D. from Nara Medical University, I decided to move to Denver, Colorado. Professor Tsubura suggested that I go to the American Medical Cancer (AMC) center. His good friend was the president of the AMC, and he knew that this would be a good opportunity for me.

In 1983, my wife Akiko, my daughter Ayako and I moved from Japan to Denver, Colorado. As one life experience was coming to a close, the adventure of a new life filled with new challenges and opportunities was waiting for me. There were both the feelings of excitement, as well as apprehension for the move I was making. But I knew my mother was right. I needed to leave Japan and I needed to leave the protection of the Ohno family name in order to find out who Yoshitaka Ohno really was.

New opportunities present themselves into our lives
When we are able to release
What no longer serves our greater good.

Yoshitaka Ohno, M.D., Ph.D.

Chapter Five

Destiny Awakening

Open your eyes and you will view life as it is
Open your mind and you discover the potential life has to offer
Open your heart and you give to life your greatest
contribution~Love

    A loom is a machine that weaves together hundreds of single threads into one whole cloth. As you look at the loom with the single, differently colored threads held inside their own separate space, it is at first difficult to imagine how these simple, thin threads are woven together to create a strong cloth with a beautiful pattern.
    Each separate experience of one's life is very much like the one single, little thread in a loom. These threads develop from every life experience we encounter because each life experience seems sometimes disassociated. The threads give the illusion of being separate from and unrelated to each other. As we evolve through each definitive experience of our life the threads we have formed interlock together and connect the events of our past to our present moment. The interconnecting of our life experiences gradually becomes the threads that effect the universal law of cause and affect and this is how our present reality is formed. Eventually, as we evolve, the threads gradually accumulate and simultaneously weave together to create a larger picture, which develops into our own personal tapestry.
    When viewed from this perspective, we can see that life is truly a form of art and we always have the artistic control to our personal design. There is an invisible energy from the universe that gently encourages our growth, guiding us and helping us to make rightful decisions that ultimately become the unfolding of

our evolution. Simultaneously, we are always in the process of becoming one with the interconnecting threads of the greater universal design. It is when our personal pattern interconnects and weaves in resonance with the greater universal design that we find ourselves following in the path of our destiny.

When we view the importance of each life experience and better understand how it affects every facet of our overall evolution, we will be able to recognize the degree of significance in the decisions we make for everything we are a part of. This realization has the potential to create a shift within our consciousness, developing a strong inner faith that becomes one with our personal structure. This faith instills within us an undying determination to move through all obstacles that seem to be in our way. The more we allow our faith to guide each and every step, the closer we come to discovering our true destiny and ultimately honoring our mission in life. There is a saying that it is within the journey, not our final destination, that we find the value of fulfillment and growth. The challenges we overcome during the journey are what causes our consciousness to grow so that we may better appreciate, not just what we have accomplished, but what we have learned along the way.

When I came to America there were tremendous challenges waiting for me. I felt as though I were crawling slowly up a very steep and rugged mountain. In the past, there were years that I couldn't see the top of the mountain because of many thick clouds that hovered over the peak. But I never gave up the climb and I never looked down. I kept my focus on conquering what lay ahead of me. So it was in America that I truly discovered myself. Everything that I had experienced before was merely the separate threads, weaving together and slowly developing a pattern of my personal tapestry. I was at last finally starting to recognize this.

To the degree of our determination
Will be the degree of our accomplishments

Yoshitaka Ohno, M.D., Ph.D.

'English 101'

Akiko, Ayako and I arrived in Denver, Colorado, in May of 1983. We rented a small apartment in Lakewood, which was about 20 minutes from AMC, (American Medical Center). On our second day in Denver, it snowed hard. I had never experienced such a snow in Japan, let alone in the month of May! As I reflect upon that May and the untimely snow, I see how the cold and bitter weather was a significant premonition of the difficulties that were ahead for me.

A few days after settling into our apartment, I started my work at the research center. My research was to be on breast cancer. I was excited about what I would learn and most importantly, what I knew I could contribute. On the plane to America, I had been filled with excitement and ambition. My mind raced with creative ideas for new cancer treatments and the prospect of a new life, driven by my enthusiasm.

However, the reality that waited for me would be harsh; I could not understand or communicate in the English language. I remembered the story of Helen Keller. Although my handicaps could be overcome in time, I was overwhelmed with the communication challenges. I gained a true respect and empathy for a woman who had overcome so much in her life through her exercise of faith and determination.

Before arriving in America I had been aware of my limitations in the English language, but I had no idea how difficult the language barrier was going to be for me to survive. I felt totally illiterate! Fortunately, my wife, Akiko, had learned the English language and could read and comprehend English fluently. I was ashamed that Akiko had to translate everything to me. When in conversation with other people, I would constantly ask her, "What are they saying to me?"

Whenever I attempted to read English, I would have to ask her, "What is the meaning of this sentence?"

Do No Harm

Every day was torture for me as I struggled to conquer this dilemma. I lost 30 pounds in the first three months, and I was down to almost 100 pounds. Shortly after, both my mother and my mother-in-law came from Japan to visit. They took one look at me and were astonished. They looked as if they did not recognize me.

"Taka!" they said, "How did this happen to you? Are you sick? Are you O.K.? You look like a skeleton!"

"I'm O.K., don't worry, everything is O.K." But everything was really not O.K., and I was not prepared to share my problem with them. I had come to America, after all, to become my own man. I was not about to tell them that I felt like a baby because I was unable to communicate. I felt like I had landed upon a different planet because everything was so different from Japan. The culture, the food, the lifestyle of the Americans, everything was so totally different. I felt like a baby who was learning to take his first steps.

My mother was very concerned for my health. She said, "Taka, this is too difficult for you, you should return to Japan. I will arrange for you and Akiko to fly back with us soon."

My mother's proposal at first seemed very tempting. But I also knew that her proposal would mean ultimate dishonor for me, because I would have to give up the entire purpose of my coming to America.

I said to her, "Mother, I cannot return to Japan now. If I come back to Japan right now, I will not be giving myself the chance to overcome my difficulties. I will not be able to achieve the promise that I made to the memory of my patients, who have died from cancer and who begged me to find a cure. I know I am meant to be here so I can work on new ideas to help cancer patients. I have made my commitment and I have to follow through with it.

"If I come back right now, I will never fulfill my promise to them. I know how difficult it is going to be for me. However, if I allow myself to give up now, I will never be able to achieve my goals. If I return to Japan, life will be easy for me. When something goes wrong, I will be protected again by the family. I will never learn to assert myself in order to grow and overcome obstacles on my own. You want to protect me because you are my mother. But it is as you and I discussed before. What will I do if something happens to you? Nobody can help me but myself. I know it is difficult for you to see my struggle, but don't you agree with me? I know that it is easy to come back to Japan, but I will be defeating the whole purpose as to why I have come to America. I cannot go back to Japan until I have accomplished my goals."

"Please trust me. Once I am successful, I will have a bright future to look forward to. I will gain confidence and I will know that there is nothing I cannot achieve for myself. I hope you understand. Please tell me that you understand!"

Nodding her head, my mother agreed, "Taka, you are correct. I want you to try your best. Even if you become sick during your struggle to succeed, then that is simply your destiny.

"I cannot say anymore, except that I trust you. This is part of your mission and you should do your best to overcome your difficulties! I really believe that you will somehow find a new solution that will lead to a cure for cancer. There is something here for you to discover, but first I know that you must discover your own inner strength. You must also learn to become the master of your talents and capabilities.

"You should not worry about anything going on in Japan. Your brother is taking care of the Ohno Hospital. You should just concentrate on learning the English language and continue your breast cancer research at AMC. I just want you to devote yourself to your own life and what you must do. Never give up, Taka! Never give up!"

My mother's words brought tears to my eyes. Once again I realized how much faith she had in me. I have been blessed to have her undying trust in me all of my life. Without her steady, positive influence, I probably would not have had the courage to go on.

Do No Harm

After the visit from my mother, I was all the more focused to conquer the English language. Even though I was so determined, I was beginning to experience difficulty sleeping and eating. My appetite was gone and I could not force myself to eat properly. My sleep was disturbed by nightmares. Many times Akiko would have to wake me up in the middle of the night.

"Taka! You have been screaming again in your sleep! You're having a nightmare!"

I was in a living hell. I was feeling the pressure of my work at AMC, and my frustration and impatience to learn English. Working on my research was much too difficult because I could not understand English. I began to suffer from hallucinations. I was imagining that the English language was attacking me. The textbooks were attacking me and saying, "Why don't you understand my meaning?

"Are you stupid? Are you a real doctor? Even though you have a license you cannot understand my meaning! You should go back to school so that you can start all over again and get your license to practice medicine!"

I quickly began to realize that before I would be able to complete my research, I had to learn the English language. My supervisor, Dr. Philip Furmanski, agreed that this is what I had to do.

"Taka, I recommend that you learn the English language before you continue your research here. Take the time you need to learn. You will have a position here when you are ready."

"Do your best and leave the rest to providence."

I went to the bookstore and purchased nine different English medical textbooks. I studied non-stop; I studied nearly 24 hours a day. I started to read the English medical books, but I was not able to comprehend anything. In the beginning I could barely read one page a day. I would read and re-read the words, trying to understand the meaning. After five months, I was able to read and understand most of my textbooks. I also began to communicate at an acceptable level. I knew that once I mastered the English language, I would want to study more than just medicine.

There were many other areas of interest that I wanted to pursue. I became very intrigued with astronomy, geology, quantum physics, molecular biology, geo-magnetism, magnetism and nutrition. I never had the opportunity to be exposed to these fields before, and I believed that the passion I had for learning was my higher self, guiding me to gain knowledge in these areas. I challenged my spirit to guide me through these new fields of knowledge. I found myself even more determined to learn English as quickly as possible.

Studying nearly 24 hours a day, my life seemed crazy. As I look back on it now, it is a wonder that I was able to survive because I was not eating nor sleeping; I was pushing my body to the point of exhaustion. If someone were to ask me today if I could work 24 hours a day, I would have to say that no one could do that. However, since I was a young man of 32 years old, I did, somehow.

My schedule seemed never ending. I worked all week, including Saturday and Sunday, as well as on holidays. I would go to AMC at 6:00 A.M., where I would read and study without a break. I would return home after work and study until 3:00 A.M. Then I would finally go to bed.

I kept up this pace for 7 years! At first, I could not comprehend my study material. Every day was a tremendous challenge for me. Studying was painfully hard work. If someone asked me to describe that time of my life, I would say it was a living hell. The more I studied, the more I struggled. Every night after I returned home from AMC, I felt defeated and depressed. I know Akiko did not find me a pleasure to live with because of my somber attitude. The first six months were extremely difficult on both of us. I was wrapped up in my own world, filled with my personal challenges, and I was not very attentive to Akiko. She generally did not want to talk to me because I was always in a bad mood. We only had one car, which I needed. She had to take the bus for shopping and running errands. Although this was an equally difficult time for her, she never once complained or said she wanted to return to Japan. She was committed to our relationship and to me. Akiko wanted us to face the challenges and overcome our difficulties together.

Eventually, the clouds at the peak of the high and rugged mountain I had been climbing began to lift. One year later I was reading 500 pages a day in *English*. I realized that *every struggle is overcome with patience*. I found that I was becoming more and more interested in my studies. I was obsessed with studying. And the more I learned, the more addicted I became to the energy and new thoughts I was receiving. It would ultimately be these subjects I had mastered that would eventually lead me into a new field of pursuit. Life was unfolding for me just as the universe had planned.

Through diligence our character becomes strengthened.

1985
News from Japan
Alzheimer disease attacks my Grandmother

Two years after Akiko and I had moved to Denver, we received sad news from my mother in Osaka.

"Taka, your grandmother has been very ill with Alzheimer's disease, and she passed away early this morning."

My mother had been taking care of her mother in our home for about five years. My mother had noticed that over time, my grandmother was losing her mental functioning. But instead of placing her in a nursing home, she had her mother come to live with her. When I had left for America, I knew that my grandmother's memory had started to fail.

"Your grandmother had progressively been getting worse. About one year ago, she became incontinent. Even though she had a portable toilet beside her bed, she could not use it. I tried to help her to the toilet every night before her bedtime, but she could not go. Finally, I found excrement on the floor."

" She started to wander out of her bed during the night and I would have to go looking for her. Sometimes she wandered miles away from our home and the police would find her. They would call me to come and get her at the police station."

My mother was very distraught as she described all of this to me. She continued, "I would ask her, Mother, where do you live? and she was not able to answer me."

"I finally had to put a diaper on her. I was not able to take care of her anymore so I had to admit her in the Ohno Hospital. However, the nurses could not take care of her either. They would leave her alone for just a moment, only to return and discover she had wandered off. The nurses said they were not able to handle her incontinence and they were not able to insure her safety.

"Last week your grandmother seemed exceptionally tired and fatigued. Although she had no fever, she had no appetite and she needed intravenous feeding. For her last three days she was in a sort of coma. When I would ask her questions, she would wake up and answer me; then she would fall back to sleep.

"I would ask her, 'Mother, do you understand me, do you know who I am?

"She would answer, Yes, you are Yoshiko.

Then one moment later, I would ask her again, Mother, who am I?

And she would answer me, "I don't know. I think you are my sister."

"Yesterday she fell into a deeper coma and she could not answer me at all. She developed pneumonia and at 3:00 this morning, your grandmother passed away."

When I heard the news, I told my mother, "Akiko and I will come back to Japan right now! I will call and arrange our travel!"

Do No Harm

I expected my mother to say that she wanted me to return home to be with her and attend my grandmother's funeral. Instead she said, "Taka, listen to me, you do not need to attend the funeral."

"What! Mother! What did you say to me? Why don't you want me to attend grandmother's funeral? What reason do you have for not wanting me to come home for grandmother's funeral?"

My mother started to cry and she said, "Taka, calm down. Of course I would like for you to come home and attend grandmother's funeral. I know how much she loved you and I know how much you loved her. Even after you and Akiko got married, she came to live with you for awhile. She always helped around the house and sometimes cooked and helped you and Akiko. I would like very much for you and Akiko to come back home but..." There was only silence on the phone.

At this point, my mother was crying.

"Mother, are you alright? Please, talk to me!"

Thirty seconds or so went by and there was still silence. Finally my mother continued.

"She left us a letter, Taka. After she died, I came back to her room to clean it up and I found a letter from her. It was totally unexpected. This letter must have been written over two years ago. It must have been very difficult for her to write this letter because of her Alzheimer's. However, she must have been very determined. She addressed it to me."

My mother read the letter to me over the phone.

Dear Yoshiko,

Thank you very much for taking care of me. Even though I am gradually losing my memory every day, you have done a nice job taking care of me. Even though my other daughter would not take care of me, you have taken care of me and loved me. I am very grateful to you.

I was so happy in my life because I had you with me. But since I have been losing my memory more everyday, I have

Yoshitaka Ohno, M.D., Ph.D.

forgotten the Japanese characters. Even though it is hard for me to understand the meanings, I decided that I must write this letter now.

I would like to say that I know I will soon not be able to recognize you. But before I die, I would like to see your Taka's face again. I know he is working very hard in America. I am sure that this time is very important for Yoshitaka.

Yoshiko! Please promise that when I die you not ask Yoshitaka to come back to attend my funeral. He does not need to attend my funeral. When he comes home to Japan, he will be able to come to my grave. But I have missed him so much and I wish I could see his face once again before I die.

By the time my mother finished the letter from my grandmother, I could not stop crying. And it was because of my grandmother's request that I did not return to Japan to attend her funeral. It is true, that when my grandmother died, I was busy with my work and study. If I had returned to Japan, I could have lost my position at the research center because there were many people there waiting to get my job. When I decided not to go back to Japan, I noticed that my focus had changed. I felt a voice within guiding me toward research in Alzheimer disease. I already knew that many people were searching for a cure for breast cancer. Even though this had been my focus, I felt strongly compelled to change the course of my research. I listened to that voice inside me, telling me to study Alzheimer's disease, because I would discover an important breakthrough.

I believed that this was the voice of "Kami" guiding me. In Japan, Kami is the spirit of Shinto. This is a philosophy that believes that Kami works to guide our lives. Kami is not God, but the spirit of God. I felt very strongly that this was the Kami energy working through me and guiding me to change the course of my research.

It was through my grandmother's passing with Alzheimer's disease that my purpose in life would once again change. I knew

Do No Harm

by now not to question the voice of my spirit, but to follow the urgings of the spiritual energy that feeds my soul.

Even with God's guidance and Kami's energy, it was very difficult for me to get started in Alzheimer's research. Unlike breast cancer, I found that there was little or no information on Alzheimer's disease. The two diseases are so completely different. When I looked up Alzheimer's disease in my textbooks, there was almost nothing to be found. I felt like I was groping in the dark. In 1983 little was known about this disease. When I asked other doctors about it, they couldn't give me any information.

I had no idea how to begin to study this disease. But I had the fighting spirit within me. I said to myself, *"It seems that nobody knows about this strange disease. There is so little research in this area. I will try my best to become knowledgeable, and if I am successful with my research, I will be able to give hope, not only to the people who have the disease, but to the family members who also suffer from its effects."*

I made a promise to myself and to my grandmother to discover something important that could lead to a cure for Alzheimer's disease.

Everything in life is for a reason.
Let us not question why certain events take place.
Rather, allow us to work through the process of each event
Knowing that eventually we will understand the 'why' of it when the time is ready.

I started to think about the other sciences that I had been studying, along with my medical studies. I was beginning to understand more about energy and the nature of the universe. There was a special commonality between astronomy, geology, quantum physics, molecular biology, geo-magnetism, magnetism and nutrition. There was something that fascinated me about these subjects and how man was directly related to all of these for survival. With what I had learned, I knew I could come up with a theory that could lead me closer to a finding a cure for Alzheimer's disease.

While I was studying, AMC was one of the first hospitals to purchase a MRI (magnetic resonance imaging). This was one of those times in my life when I was in the right place at the right time. While working with the MRI, I learned how to diagnose the brain of Alzheimer's disease patients. The only difference I could detect in a brain of a person with Alzheimer's disease was that its structures are reduced from the normal size. This is really the only way to distinguish the difference. The MRI could not diagnose memory loss, which is the major symptom of Alzheimer's disease.

Even today, with new technology in diagnostics, Alzheimer's can not be diagnosed accurately because it resembles other forms of dementia. The diagnosis of Alzheimer's is only differential, after the process of elimination. In fact, only from an autopsy can Alzheimer's be accurately diagnosed. One interesting observation seen in an autopsy is the formation of plaques around nerve fibers, as well as tangled nerve fibers. These formations will eventually shut down cognitive functioning. This is the most common factor seen in brains of Alzheimer's victims.

As I continued to study the brain, an amazing thought entered my mind. The brain consists mostly of water. Our body is made up of 70% of water, but the brain is made up of almost 90% water. The more I thought about this, the more I realized the importance of the quality of the water in our brain. If the water in the brain is in any way contaminated, it will affect brain structure and function. Surely, with the brain being made up of 90% water, there had to be some connection between water in the brain and how Alzheimer's disease develops. I was convinced that this was a very important link. I also realized that there is much information about the major influence of water and magnetism on human anatomy and physiology.

I often wondered why I was led to study so many different scientific fields. I had only known that I was drawn by a very

Do No Harm

strong urge. If I had not studied so many fields, I would never have understood the important interrelationship of water and magnetism in our bodies, which led me to my theory on Alzheimer's disease. Many times people would ask me why I was studying so many different fields at the same time. I could not answer them because I really did not have the answer. I only felt that I was being guided by some invisible force, which was leading me to discover something important. The more I studied Alzheimer disease, the more I realized that I was on the right path to discovering the cause of Alzheimer's disease and how to successfully treat it.

Even after I realized how important good water is for the brain, I could not figure out how improving the quality of the water in the brain could improve cognitive functioning. I studied and struggled with different concepts on increasing cognitive functioning. Then I found a paper written by Dr. Raymond Damadian, who had been a candidate for the Nobel Prize. He had studied the water in cells by using the MRI to distinguish the difference between a cancer cell and a normal cell. He found in his study using rats as test subjects that the cancer cell's water is so much more aggressive than a normal cell.

Under the MRI, a normal cell's water is organized and moves in an orderly flow. However, the cancer cell's water is very aggressive and disorganized, and its movement is rapid and random, as well as disorganized. In 1973, Dr. Damadian furthered his research using human cancer patients to check the water movement inside of the cell. He concluded again that the water in a cancer cell is much more aggressive and disorganized than the water movement in a normal cell. However, under a MRI, even the water in cancer cells will be organized.

I came up with an interesting question. If a MRI could be used for diagnosis to determine differences in cell water, why couldn't some form of treatment be created that could duplicate MRI effect on keeping cell water organized in its movement.

I know that when a patient is lying on a MRI bed, the water molecules in tissues are organized during the magnetic imaging procedure. But when the MRI is removed, water in cancer cells returns to a disorganized pattern and aggressive movement. I wondered if the MRI could somehow be used for treatment since it corrected the movement of the water inside the cell.

Looking at the structure of a cell during the MRI process, the magnetic influence of the MRI draws an electron, which then keeps the structure of the cell organized and stable. But without magnetic influence, an electron can be lost, which returns the cell to disorganization. Even though Dr. Damadian's paper had been published over 15 years before, nobody had researched the concept of his idea of water movement within the human cell and the correlation with homeostasis. Even though his findings were exciting, they had not sparked enough interest for further investigation.

Through my studies of magnetization and water, which supported the research that Dr. Damadian had done, I got the idea that if a water was permanently magnetized, it would definitely be worthy of investigation to see its affect on treating diseases such as Alzheimer's and cancer. Through all of my studies, water and magnetism were the most common factors in creating a balance in the Universe and on Earth, as well as homeostasis in our bodies.

Since I studied Astronomy, I realized how rare the Earth is in the solar system. Even though there are nine planets in the solar system, the only living planet is Earth. Water is the reason for life on Earth. The first life was born in the water. After billions of years, organisms then moved to occupy land. But even with this advance in evolution, all life form still was composed of mostly water.

The human body has the same percentage of water as the Earth. The Earth is made up of 70% water and our body is also 70% water. When I studied molecular biology, I learned that our cells also consist of 70% water. If the quality of the water in our cells is not good, then our health cannot be good.

Geomagnetism also influences the behavior of water. Ocean water is affected by the magnetism of the moon. The water in

Do No Harm

our bodies is also affected by the magnetic influence of the moon in the same way. When the ocean is at high tide, our body water is also at high tide, due to the magnetic influence of the moon. And the level of energy in our bodies also increases when the moon is full. It is generally known that there is an easier birth of a baby when there is a full moon and a high tide. This is because the baby is contained in the mother's amniotic fluid, and when the amniotic fluid is at "high tide", the birth is easier. On the other hand, when there is a low tide, our body energy is low. Even though we are not consciously aware of the impact of the magnetic influence from the moon, we are none the less affected by the phases of the moon. If we learn to take advantage of this natural phenomenon in how we create our life style, we can live longer and healthier lives.

My knowledge of geology has helped me recognize the various geographical zones and the different energies in each one. The Earth has many different layers, or grids, that vibrate on different frequency levels in accordance with a specific area. We all have traveled to places where we felt very serene and comfortable, or more energized being in that geographical area. One example is Sedona, Arizona. Sedona has many vortexes that contain healing energy. Several thousands of visitors come to Sedona every year to experience the calming, energizing, and healing vibrations. Many people even experience life changes, physical healing, or receive general enlightenment that stays with them long after they have left the vortex area.

There are also areas that have a negative impact upon us. These are generally areas in which we choose not to live or visit because of the poor energy we receive. There is a strong relationship between the place and the spirit that flows. Because some places have a strong energy field, the water in those places has a very strong energy. Geo-magnetism determines the Earth's magnetism. If geo-magnetism is decreased, our joints become stiff, we get headaches and we have much less energy. When we are provided with the right amount of magnetism, we once again come back to a state of equilibrium with a healthier body.

Yoshitaka Ohno, M.D., Ph.D.

In Quantum physics, I recognized that it is the force of electrons orbiting the cell that creates energy. Once an electron is lost and is no longer paired, we become sick. Free radicals form when an electron is lost, and a cell looks to replace it by taking an electron from another cell. Thus, another free radical is formed. If there is a way to return lost electrons, energy will be restored and homeostasis returned.

Through the combination of all of my research in these separate fields, I came to the realization of how important magnetization is to organize water in our cells to increase its energy field and return to healthful functioning. The organized cells have a balanced number of electrons in pairs, but disorganized cells have unbalanced electrons. I concluded that if we consumed permanently magnetized water, the magnetization would give the electron back to the cells and, thus eliminate free radicals. This would definitely change the course of many diseases.

But how can an electron be given back to disorganized water within the cell? This would require that the water be permanently magnetized. Artificially magnetized water does not last for more than 6-8 hours after it is magnetized. I knew that if water could influence cell structure and function, it would have to be naturally magnetized so it would not lose its magnetization.

I discussed this idea with a specialist of magnetization. I asked him, "Have you ever heard of a naturally, permanently magnetized water?"

He answered me, "Are you silly? There is no such thing! I don't think you understand the principles of magnetization. I recommend that you study more about magnetization!"

I talked about my idea to other MRI researchers. I told them, *"Many diseases are caused by disorganized water in the cells. In order to get from disorganized water to organized water, we would have to lie down on a MRI forever. If we had a way other than the MRI to give the body a permanent magnetization, then I believe that we would be able to successfully treat many diseases."*

Do No Harm

One researcher told me, "Your idea is nonsense because Alzheimer's disease is caused by metals such as aluminum, not contamination of the water inside the cell. Even though your idea about free radicals may be correct, you are not going to find a water that is naturally magnetized. I have never heard of permanently magnetized water."

I was not discouraged by the opinions of the researchers who advised me. I knew from my past experience that most people questioned me and they thought me crazy because of my different views. I also knew that I needed to continue my pursuit of this theory. The more people made fun of my ideas, the more it motivated me to prove them wrong. I continued my research in Alzheimer's disease. In 1989, I received an award for my contribution. Princess Yasamin A. Gakareen, the Honorable President of the Alzheimer's Association International, presented the Humanitarian Award for Excellence to me. This was in addition to the award I received from the Colorado Alzheimer's Association for my research.

As I continued in my struggle to find a cure for Alzheimer's disease, I searched for magnetized water in America. I knew that in order for water to have a permanent magnetization, there would have had to be a very unusual geomagnetic phenomenon. I began to spend much of my time looking for a source of naturally magnetized water. I studied the history of geographical eras throughout the world, trying to find an area that might contain this special, unique water.

I had much faith that the miracle I was searching for was waiting somewhere for me. I never doubted it for a moment. I decided it was now time for me to return once again to Japan. I had not been able to find the magnetized water I was looking for in America, so perhaps I needed to return to my home country and search for it there. I had left years earlier for a completely different reason. Before, I felt as though I had to leave Japan to find my independence. Now, I was returning home to hopefully find what I did not have the eyes to see before. As always, the natural forces of the universe were guiding me and directing me.

Yoshitaka Ohno, M.D., Ph.D.

Now, I was able to understand and feel this energy, and I allowed it to work with me as I walked in my faith.

> *Stand still for a moment and reflect upon your life*
> *What does your personal tapestry look like?*
> *Open your eyes, your mind, and your heart and know*
> *That you have the power within to design your life*
> *To match your dreams and desires.*

Chapter Six

Returning Home

As you place trust in your Self ~
And you are honest with your Self ~
You nurture the most important relationship you'll ever have ~
The relationship of Self.

After seven years in Denver, Colorado I knew it was time to return home to Osaka, Japan. Even though we were excited and looking forward to reuniting with our families, there was at the same time an element of apprehension. There is a saying, *"You can never go home again"* meaning that things change and the memories you carry in your mind are not always the reality you return to.

I had worked hard to learn and conquer the English language. I had once again overcome many obstacles while simultaneously pursuing the search for my purpose. And now I was returning home feeling victorious from what I had set out to do. I had learned that I could make it on my own without the protection of the Ohno family shielding me from the outside world. I had accomplished a lot, but I was aware that my real work had yet to begin. Through my studies and the research I pursued while I was in Denver, I was able to gain a true vision of what I wanted to do. I was determined that my ideas about the importance of water and its effect on health would be my focus. I had to search for a source of the water I knew would support my theory.

It takes over 12 hours to fly from Denver to Japan, and that gives one a great deal of time to think. I thought about my ideas and I wondered if the Japanese Medical Society was still as conservative as it used to be. I talked to people on the plane and explained my ideas about the importance of water in relation to

Yoshitaka Ohno, M.D., Ph.D.

health. They liked my idea and I felt hopeful. I had a feeling of optimism and was looking forward to getting home.

My family and I were tired as we made it through customs. With the time change and the long flight, it felt as though we had traveled for days. We were looking forward to being picked up by my brother, Yoshioki, and going home for a long rest.

We could hear a lot of people cheering as we walked through the gate. There was a lot of activity going on. It seemed like there must have been a celebrity or dignitary expected, as a crowd of people waited anxiously outside. When we walked through the gate we were stunned to see all of our family, friends and several people we didn't know saying,"Welcome home, Dr. Ohno and family! Welcome home!"

I was so surprised to see such a big crowd, and everyone was so happy to see us! We were speechless, not having anticipated the crowd of people and the special greeting they were giving us.

Finally, out of the crowd, I saw my mother. I heard her say, "Welcome back, Taka!" And my brother Yoshioki appeared saying, "Welcome back, Taka!"

We greeted everyone and tried to smile and thank them for coming to welcome us home.

It seemed like an hour before we were able to make our way to the car and home to Osaka. During the ride home, I asked my mother why there were so many people at the airport to welcome us home. She said that my uncle, Yorioki Hamuro, had arranged for our special welcome because we had been gone for seven long years. My uncle, Yorioki Hamuro, is the Chief Priest of the Kasuga Shrine in Nara, Japan. He has a very kind heart and I have always admired him.

When we arrived at my mother's house, I realized how good it was to be home. All of my favorite Japanese foods had been prepared for our return. It seemed like it was a special Japanese holiday! We didn't even notice a jet lag as we settled in to visit and reunite with our family. It was especially good to be with my mother and my brother again. I began to share my experience in America and explained that although I had missed

Do No Harm

them very much, it was important to me to leave Japan so I could pursue my dream.

After a wonderful meal, my wife Akiko and my children went to bed. I stayed up to visit more with my mother and my brother. It felt so good to be with them in the quiet of our home. As my mother poured hot tea, she looked at me and said,

"Taka, life has presented you with so many challenges since the time you have been very young, yet you have been successful in meeting all of these challenges. I think learning English and your research at AMC in Denver have been your greatest challenges so far. When I saw you and the look of pride in your face when you arrived today, I affirmed to myself that you have conquered your toughest difficulty!"

My brother nodded in agreement. Then I said, "Thank you very much mother. Thank you very much brother.

"It is because you have shown your trust and your faith in me that I have been able to conquer my difficulties! If you did not trust me, I would not have been successful! You see, if I had stayed in Japan, no matter what I would have done, I would still have been under the Ohno umbrella. I had to go to another country and away from the Ohno family to discover my true strength. It was a challenge, but I am proud of my accomplishments and I have grown into a stronger person. I know now that I can survive on my own."

"Mother, I appreciate you for supporting me in my decision to stay in America to prove what I could do. I know you are very wise and you were aware that you needed to let me face the adversity of another country, another language and another culture."

"Taka, there is a saying, love well, whip well. Sometimes a parent has to allow their children to undertake certain difficulties even though it hurts to watch them struggle. This is how I knew you would come into your own. You were an indulged child. I could see that unless you were presented with challenges in your life, you would not discover your compassionate heart. You were a late bloomer, but the late fruit keeps well! You needed to extend more effort than the normal person in order to come into your own. Learning to apply effort to overcome your difficulties has given you the opportunity to become compassionate and to become a better person. Now you are a person of honor. Because you have given the effort of ten people in order to be successful, I know that you will have good fortune in the future because you have learned the value of effort."

"Taka, I believe a human being's life span is determined at birth. Some people are meant to die when they are only 10 years of age; some people die when they turn 100 years of age. But even though the life span is already determined at birth, if a person lives life to the fullest and puts in his or her best effort, a longer life is possible. Destiny provides an 80 percent factor in life and effort adds 20 percent."

"When babies are born, the genes they have received from their parents determine the DNA of their bodies. So that, you may wonder, how can effort or one's thinking have an impact on the life span? If you drink too much, or if you take drugs or smoke, then you are affecting the quality of your health. This will affect your life span. Many people abuse their bodies with alcohol or with smoking, and if they get cancer from abusing their bodies, they will not take responsibility for what happens to them. Many times they complain and ask God why He gave them cancer. Even though they had control over how to take care of themselves, they refused to take responsibility for their actions."

"The quality of human life most often depends on how people take care of themselves. It is important to give appreciation and to think with an appreciative heart. The mind has a direct correlation to the health of the body, and the spirit is enhanced when we take care of ourselves. This is the mind-body-spirit relationship I believe in."

"Taka! You are fortunate that you have experienced so much. You have learned what a person is capable of doing when he puts his mind to it. You have also learned empathy and effort. It has not been your fortune but your misfortune that has

Do No Harm

helped you grow. Your experience will help you in the future because you are meant to help people in a humanitarian way. Never forget what you have gone through and God will always help you and guide you along your path. God will always be there to help guide you!"

"Mother! I understand what you have told me and I will always remember your words of wisdom. I believe there has always been an invisible force, a powerful energy guiding me. I already know what I need to do to accomplish my goals to help people."

I discussed the theory I had formed while doing my research at AMC. I explained to them my ideas regarding the MRI and the magnetization process of the body while under the influence of a MRI.

"Yoshioki, why could the way an MRI works not be used for treatment?

"I suppose, Taka, that with the MRI the body is exposed to a steady magnetization, but after the MRI is removed, then the body returns to its normal state without magnetism."

"Yoshioki, what I think is that with the MRI, the body receives such strong magnetization that the water in the body becomes more organized so diagnosis can be achieved. However, after the patient is exposed to the MRI, the water resorts back to a disorganized situation. I believe if we keep the water in the cells organized with magnetization, this can be used as treatment for many diseases!"

"Taka, your idea makes sense. However, it is impossible to keep a strong magnetization in water forever. It is impossible to be under a MRI forever. Because this is not possible, then your idea is not very workable. Permanent exposure to a MRI is not good for our bodies and it is not a practical situation. The only thing that makes sense is a magnetized substance taken into the body."

"You are exactly right, Yoshioki. That is exactly my idea and one of the reasons why I have returned home! I have made up my mind to find a natural source that produces naturally magnetized water!"

"But that is much easier said than done, Taka. How do you plan to find a naturally magnetized water?"

"Yoshioki, I believe I wouldn't have gotten this idea which I believe has been given to me, if the water wasn't somewhere to be found!"

My mother listened to Yoshioki and I talking about my idea. She sipped her tea and asked me, "Taka, what will you do now to earn a living now that you are home? Will you return to the pathology department in Nara or will you come back to Ohno Hospital?"

I had wondered myself just where I would go and how I would earn a living. I could not answer promptly because I had yet to look into the situations available at the hospital and at the pathology department in Nara. I was anxious about working at the hospital because Yoshioki was the director there. I didn't want to cause friction with Yoshioki by working there, and both my mother and Yoshioki were of the same mind. I had been away from clinical studies at Nara Hospital for nearly seven years, and I felt my absence was too long for me to try to catch up with what they were researching in pathology. Also, it had been nearly 11 years since I had practiced medicine.

My main interest was now in MRI and disease. But, if I wanted to study this at the Nara Hospital, I would have to go to the radiology department. Aside from my study of the MRI and courses in medical school, I had no advanced professional education or training in radiology. I wanted to continue with my investigation of magnetization and its influence on health, but I also had to be very careful whom I told. I was worried that if I told my idea to a medical professor, he would steal the idea.

My mother said, "I don't want you to go to a major research center because I believe your idea will be taken from you before you can prove the results and publish the findings in your name. I don't want to see you go through what happened to Dr. Maruyama. He had such a creative idea, but both Japan's

Do No Harm

Medical Society and the pharmacological industry crushed his idea. Since you are not a graduate of Tokyo University, even though you publish this work, there will be no one who will listen to you. If you had graduated from Tokyo University, then I would definitely recommend that you publish your ideas."

Mother looked at me very seriously "My honest opinion, Taka, is that you should keep this idea to yourself until the time is ready. First you must find a water source that is permanently magnetized, then you must do clinical studies to get evidence that your idea works. Just keep in mind, Taka, that even if you prove the validity of your idea and publish your findings, you may not want to do it in Japan

We discussed at length my idea and how I believed Alzheimer's disease, cancer and even diabetes patients would benefit from the type of water I was looking for. I explained to my mother and Yoshioki why artificially magnetized water would not be effective.

My mother questioned me again about what I wanted to do. She did not want me to pursue magnetized water studies in Japan because of its medical politics. I would have to decide what I could do to make my living since doing magnetized water studies at the Ohno Hospital or at the Nara pathology department were not reasonable opportunities for me to pursue.

My mother looked at me very seriously and said, "Taka, I have given your situation a great deal of thought. Our family business, the Ohno Company, needs someone in charge that can handle all of the affairs. My opinion is that since you have been away for so long, you should change your focus for awhile and learn the family business so you can help protect our assets."

I was astonished to hear what my mother wanted me to do, "What! I am not a businessman! What do I know about handling business? Other than helping out at the hospital as a director years ago, I have never taken care of business in my life! I have worked hard in developing a creative idea and I have dreamed of being able to continue my research and to find a way to help people and prevent disease!"

"But Taka, you are not in a position to work in the medical field here. The only thing left for you to consider is to become a businessman and run the Ohno Company business. It is very important that you learn to become a businessman to help our family. You may find that you are interested in this area of work and even find satisfaction in it."

I could not disagree with my mother. She had always trusted and encouraged me, especially in times of great challenge. The least I could do was to help the family in any way I possibly could. I sat pondering the situation and finally I said, "O.K.! I agree with you. Even though I have no previous experience in the family business, I will give you my word that I will try my best."

Everything had changed for me within a matter of moments. One minute I was excited about my vision to find a magnetized water source, and the next minute my mother is convincing me to work in the family business. The two worlds couldn't have been further apart. But what was I to do? I couldn't disappoint my mother or my brother. After all, they had given me their personal support, love, and patience. Since I had been away from home so long, all I could do was agree with my mother and take the responsibility I had to the family. But I wondered how I would do and if my heart would be into this new venture. I also wondered when and how I would be able to pursue my dream.

Do No Harm

Yoshitaka Ohno
President
Ohno Company

I felt like a fish out of water. I awoke the very next morning and made my way to downtown Osaka where our business offices were located. I went to my office and sat at my desk. I did nothing all day. I did nothing, that is, but feel miserable and think to myself, *Why did I go to America? To become a businessman? Why did I study so hard in Colorado to learn the MRI? Why do I feel so defeated?* I felt very depressed and everything seemed gloomier as time went by.

I would awake at six A.M. and get dressed in a business suit. I would take the train by seven. I was in the office by eight. Every day, I sat down in my chair and looked for something to do. Even though I had many staff people and my name was on the door as 'President ', I felt useless. I was just a figure-head and the staff resented me for being there. If I had some knowledge or interest in the business activities, I am sure it would have felt more satisfying. But I had no interest in business and to work at this job with a glorified title bothered me. Again, as during so many times in my life, I felt as though I was trapped.

My days were mentally stressful as I attempted to cope with my depressed state. Gradually, I became like many other Japanese executives and began stopping for a drink every day after work. I didn't go home many days until after midnight because I had been drinking all evening. I was drinking every day. I was not proud of myself, but I couldn't figure out how to cope with a new situation I was once again finding myself in.

Yoshitaka Ohno, M.D., Ph.D.

Tsutomu, my friend
You continue to help me, even now.

During this time something happened that changed my life again when an old friend called me.

"Taka! Are you coming with us for our yearly visit to pay honor to Tsutomu Okamoto?"

"Yes, of course I will attend," I promptly replied.

When I said yes, I immediately remembered my good friend's face and the memory I had of him. He was a very handsome man with an athletic body. He almost had not seemed Japanese; he did not have the typical Japanese features. He was almost 6 feet tall. Tsutomu was always a good friend. When people met him, they were immediately attracted by his personality. Every body liked Tsutomu. Fondly, I remembered his nickname was "*Tsu-Bou.*

I had known Tsu-Bou since grade school. When we were in elementary school he was an excellent student and always received the highest grades. My grades were not nearly as good as his were. He was the most popular student in our class. After finishing elementary school, we were separated and went to different junior high schools. But even though we were in different schools we remained good friends.

I went to Kurume Medical University, which is in southern Japan. Tsutomu went to Kansai Gakuin University, which is in the center of Japan. But whenever I would return to Osaka, we would get together and play a round of golf. Our relationship never changed; we were always the best of friends. Tsutomu always raised my spirits and made me feel good to be in his presence. I had always honored him as a friend for life.

When I had decided to go to Denver, Colorado, Tsutomu held a farewell golf party for me with our closet friends, Susumu Araki and Hiroshi Satoo. We all had known each other since Fuzoku Ikeda Shogakko Elementary School. We called ourselves the Fusho Group. It was a huge party to send me off in

Do No Harm

style. Tsutomu also arranged another party for my family as well.

Suddenly, my pleasant thoughts of Tsutomu were dimmed with the memory of the 1985 tragedy I have tried so often to forget. There had been 240 passengers in the airplane. No one could have imagined their fate as they flew over Mt. Fuji on a routine flight from Tokyo to Osaka. From the accounts of the investigation, the airplane had started to swing erratically. The airplane suddenly lost one wing! The pilot had no way of controlling the ill-fated plane. Passengers screamed as the plane tilted at a high angle and dropped at a high speed directly for a mountain. The pilot radioed for help, over and over, but there was nothing that could be done as the control tower listened helplessly. In a matter of only 10 seconds, it was over. The airplane crashed into the mountain leaving, miraculously, one lone survivor, a stewardess.

One of the victims, Kyu Sakamoto, was a famous Japanese popular singer. His record, "Sukiyaki", became a big hit in the U.S. 20 years earlier.

I heard the news in Denver and could not believe my ears. Tsutomu had just been here recently to visit my family and me and help us out. He had come to Colorado on business and to meet with former President Ford in Vail with 20 other business associates. During his stay in Vail, he contacted me and we were able to meet for a game of golf. Tsutomu had been very concerned about me because I had lost 30 pounds and he had hoped to get me out to cheer me up.

When he came to visit Akiko and me in our apartment, he was surprised to see me driving a junk car. Tsutomu asked me, "Taka, why don't you buy a better car?"

"I cannot afford a better car now, Tsutomu."

"Well, I will tell your brother, Yoshioki, about your situation and have him ask your family to buy you a better car!"

After Tsutomu talked to my mother and my brother, my mother sent us the money to buy a new car. In addition to being my best friend, Tsutomu became my benefactor.

Yoshitaka Ohno, M.D., Ph.D.

It saddened me so much to hear of his death. What made this even worse was that just before the plane crash, Tsutomu had made plans to come back to visit us in Colorado. Instead, he decided to postpone the trip and go to Tokyo on business. He died on the return flight to Osaka. What if he came to Colorado instead? Would he still be alive today? This thought was always on my mind.

All of my life he had been such a good friend. I couldn't believe he was gone so quickly, and I couldn't imagine someone with such a kind heart to die in the way he did. I asked God, "Why did you let him die?" I wondered why so many people I had cared for so deeply had died an untimely death. But the anger I felt was not going to help Tsutomu return to me. I would miss him so much and I would never see him again. I was not able to return to Japan for his funeral, but now I could at least visit his grave.

It was a cloudy day. The sky was holding back the rain, as if God didn't want my visit to be disturbed. I found Tsutomu's grave in his family plot. There were nearly 30 of us there to pay our respects and honor his memory. We said our private prayers as we each held our fond memories of him in our hearts. After awhile, the group started to break up and many had wandered away from the gravesite. I felt a hesitation to leave and so I lingered there by myself. Memories of our deep friendship, our laughter, the dreams we had shared, how he had been there to help me in a time of need flooded my mind.

All of a sudden, I felt as though he were standing beside me. I looked around and almost expected to see him there. The feeling of him close by seemed to be so real to me. Then suddenly, I heard his words, "Taka! Welcome back! I am so glad to see you. I haven't seen you in such a long time!"

"Thank you, Taka. I am so happy that you have come to visit me. You were always my best friend and I have missed you. I knew that someday you would come and visit me here."

It was as though he were alive and standing right beside me. It felt so incredibly real. It seemed like yesterday that we had

Do No Harm

my farewell party before I left for America. And it seemed like yesterday that he and I had played golf in Vail. I rubbed the tears from my eyes and shook my head, unable to leave.

Then he continued, "Taka, I was happy to help you and your wife get a new car. I was worried about you then and I was happy to help you out."

I asked Tsutomu, "Why didn't you come back to visit me in Denver like you planned? If you had come back, you would not have been in the plane crash!"

"Because even though our group had decided to go back to Vail then, I declined because I didn't want to leave my wife behind again."

I stood there wondering where the fine lines of destiny and the decisions that humans make begin and end. I wondered how much control we really have on what happens to us in our lives. I wondered if Tsutomu had made a different decision and had not been on that ill-fated plane, would he have been alive today? Was it Tsutomu's fate to have died that day anyway, some other way? All of these questions were running through my head. And here I was standing at his grave, communicating with his spirit. Suddenly, my thoughts were interrupted as Tsutomu continued with his dialogue. "Taka, What are you doing to yourself?"

" Don't you feel shame for yourself? I see you drinking every day and losing your purpose. What happened to your vision and your promises to the people you wanted to help? Where is your good heart, Taka? Where is your humanitarian spirit?"

His words stunned me. I looked around and found I was all alone. Physically alone but spiritually connected with Tsutomu. He was giving me a verbal beating and one I clearly deserved. He continued to speak to me as the sky darkened and the heavy clouds above began to rumble with thunder. I started to feel drops of rain gently fall on my face. The raindrops gathered and mingled with the teardrops that were already on my cheeks. In this unreal moment, I continued to remain silent and listen intensely to him.

I realized my visit today to his grave had been for a definite purpose. Nothing in life is by accident, I decided. Tsutomu's death had not been unavoidable; all of life is by design. Tsutomu had come to give love and to spread his friendship and his joy to many people who had needed him. Death was not going to keep his genuine spirit from reaching out to help me today. So, I stayed and I listened, and Tsutomu continued,

"Taka, have you already forgotten your promise, your mission to help people? If you lose your spirit and your commitment to help people, God will definitely be upset with you.

"Taka! Are you listening? You must quit working in your family business and return to your research! This is your true destiny. Don't give up now!

"If you stay in Japan you will lose your humanitarian spirit! Japan is not good for you because you lose yourself within your family. You will lose your passion for life and your compassion for mankind. If you fulfill your destiny and find the water you are looking for, you must return to America to continue your research."

In a moment, everything occupying my mind shifted. Tsutomu's words rang loud and clear within my soul. He was right. I had let my fighting spirit dwindle by working in the family business, where I had no interest or expertise. I knew that I must wake up to the realization that my spirit was committing suicide by not following my dream, my ideals.

I believe God guided me that day and helped me once again by acting through my friend Tsutomu. God knew I would listen to my long time friend. I think God had been trying to reach me so many times before I started to lose my way, but I was not listening. I did, however, listen to the spirit of my dear and cherished friend. I knew that a miracle had just happened and I was once again reminded of my destiny. Every time I think I am controlling my life, I realize I am wrong. God guides each life.

Do No Harm

God guides us with a gentle hand and points the direction, but we need to apply the effort. Effort is what makes the difference as to how our life turns out.

Tsutomu died at the young age of 35. That was his destiny. We always think that we are the center of the universe, but we are wrong. Our lives are decided by God, and God created the miracle to transfer Tsutomu's spirit and energy to me that day so that I would finally wake up out of my deep, dark depression.

The rain was falling heavily now and I noticed that I was getting soaked. I had no idea how long I had been standing there by Tsutomu's grave. I vowed to Tsutomu and I vowed once again to the patients and the many people I had made promises to that I would continue with my work. The rain seemed so cleansing, as if it were washing away what was destroying my life. It was bathing me with a rebirth of spirit. The spirit I had forgotten about and was replacing with alcohol. I knew I no longer needed alcohol.

I spent many days after my experience at Tsutomu's grave thinking about my values. I had always focused on giving hope to people and making a profit was never important to me. I always wanted to devote myself to helping people without my ego getting in the way. Too many people allow their ego to get in the way of their true spiritual nature, by focusing too much on money and the materialistic part of their life.

I believe Tsutomu's energy had transferred to me that day in front of his grave a good spiritual energy that gave me strength. There is a spiritual energy that transfers from generations of ancestors and through people who have strong connections. I always felt that spiritual energy had transferred to my mother from my father when he died. She gained a new strength for the new responsibilities she had to deal with after his death.

I believed very strongly that because I had a humanitarian heart and not a heart in need of material rewards, I would find the water I knew existed that would lead me to the answers I was seeking. I concentrated on my gratitude for the life I was being given, because I knew that only with a heart filled with gratitude would I get to where I needed to go. I told of my experience at Tsutomu's grave to my mother.

My mother cried as I described what had happened to me. She had known Tsutomu since he was a young child. After she stopped crying she said to me, "Taka, I think Tsutomu came to you so that you would know that you must devote your life to research. I think that you have been miserable attempting to work in the family business. You have too good a heart to work in business. You are generous and business is a greedy world that will contaminate you with other greedy people.

"I agree with Tsutomu that you should quit working in the family business and go back to pursuing your work. You need to study more geology so you can learn where to find regions where there has been a strong impact on the earth from the atmosphere. Then maybe this is where you will find this special water you have had visions about. If you concentrate on your spiritual energy and allow it to guide you, Taka, you will find the water source. It is waiting for you, I know it!

I feel you should go to the Kasuga Shrine in Nara to see your uncle Yoriaki. You know he is the Chief Priest and he is very knowledgeable about water. Much of what he writes and lectures about is water and nature keeping mankind in balance. He may be able to direct you to different areas in Japan to search for your water."

The next day I went to Kasuga Shrine, in Nara to visit mother's brother, the Chief Priest. Until he was 50 years old, he was a very famous doctor. He quit the medical field, where he specialized in cleft palate corrective surgery, to become a Shinto priest. He had devoted himself to medicine because of a special healing he received when he was a young medical student.

He had been suffering from tuberculosis and was told that he could expect to live only three more months. He was told to prepare himself to face this horrible tragedy. And this he did. Believing he was going to die, he turned himself over to his fate, and awaited the end of his life on earth.

Do No Harm

One day he read a book that explained that man does not determine his life but that God determines man's life. These words had made a profound impact upon him, and he wept with the realization that he needed to release himself completely into God's hands. He wept for hours and upon finishing the book, he discovered that his tuberculosis was gone. A miracle had taken place in his body and he had been completely healed.

He vowed to devote his life to helping people in the way God directed him. As a medical student, he saw many cleft palate patients enter the hospital. At that time, there was little knowledge or success in performing a successful procedure. This was a long and delicate operation. Many patients left in worse condition because an operation had not been successful.

My uncle searched for new ways to perfect this procedure. Finally, he met a Japanese doctor who specialized in cleft palate corrective surgery. He taught my uncle all that he knew. After much training and practice, my uncle opened up his own clinic specializing in this procedure. His surgeries were successful and his reputation grew throughout Japan. He specialized in infants and children. He performed nearly 1000 operations, and each one generally took over seven hours. I visited my uncle when I was in medical school and I attempted to help him in one of his operations. I was amazed at how many hours he was able to concentrate and work on his patient. I asked him how he was able to do it.

"I concentrate on my compassion for the young patient I am operating on. I focus on my spirituality and the spiritual energy of the patient. There is a connection between my spiritual energy and the patient's. The trust between my patient and me, and the trust we both have in God makes the operation a success. If there is not mutual trust and faith, then the operation would not be successful."

After almost 30 years, my uncle decided to leave medicine and become a priest. As he had been guided to become a doctor and specialize in a certain field, he also had been guided to change his vocation.

I told my uncle my story about what happened to me at Tsutomu's grave. I explained to him about the MRI and my studies in all of the different scientific fields while I was in America. Most importantly, I shared with him my ideas about magnetization and my dream to find a miracle water that could change sickness to wellness.

"Taka, I have always known how important the quality of water is for the human body. Usually a person becomes sick because the quality of the water in their body is bad; whereas if the water in their body is good, they experience steady health. Our life depends upon the quality of the water we give it."

"Kasuga Shrine was built over 1000 years ago in this area because this is a very special place with very special energy. This is why the shrine was built on this land. But now the water at the shrine is not as good as it used to be. I challenge you to find a good source of quality of water. It must be free of chemicals and toxins, and it must have a special energy that is not found in any other water. Then, it will definitely be beneficial to people's health."

After talking to my uncle, I crystallized in my mind what I had to do. I would devote my life to searching for a good water source.

Chapter Seven

The Living Waters of Japan's Ancient Magnetic Mountain

Throughout the history of religions and legends, two things are always held sacred – mountain and water.

The mountain is home to the gods of mythology, and where Abraham, Moses and Mohammed sought and found God. Water has purified and healed. It is the eternal symbol of life.

Destiny Leads Me to a Tofu Restaurant in Kyoto And My Search is Over

On a cold day one year after I returned to Japan, I decided to visit Kyoto. Kyoto is one of the most popular Japanese tourist attractions. It was the home of ancient Emperors and is still one of the most beautiful cities in the world. I went to Kyoto for no particular reason, other than to relax and enjoy.

The cold wind had set in under my skin, and hot tea and tofu was what I needed to warm up. Being unfamiliar with Kyoto, I asked the taxi driver, "I am from Osaka and have just arrived. Can you take me to a restaurant that has the best tofu?"

"I know just the place!" he said.

As we were driving along I expected him to deliver me to an expensive restaurant in one of the more exclusive parts of Kyoto. But when he stopped in front of a small building that resembled a run down house rather than a good restaurant, I asked him if he had misunderstood my request. I had an unpleasant feeling

Yoshitaka Ohno, M.D., Ph.D.

when I looked at the old structure. I sat in the backseat, hesitating to get out of the taxicab.

"Here we are! This is the restaurant you wanted!" the cab driver said.

"Are you sure they have good tofu here? This doesn't look very promising to me!"

"You said you wanted good tofu and this is by far the best tofu in all of Kyoto, and maybe all of Japan! Every taxi driver knows about this place and they would have brought you here as well. I know this place is not fancy, but if you really want the 'best' tofu, I have brought you to the right place."

"What makes the tofu so special here? What makes it different from the other good restaurants in Kyoto?" I asked.

"I have no idea. I just know it is the best. Ask anyone in Kyoto. But if you prefer, I can take you to another restaurant if that makes you feel more comfortable," he offered.

"No, you don't have to take me to another place. You have my curiosity now by your high recommendation, and I would very much like to try the tofu here and taste the 'best' tofu in Kyoto!"

I paid the cab driver and went into the small restaurant. I was very surprised to see that the place was packed. I would have an hour wait before I was seated. After the waitress guided me to my table, I scanned the menu she had given me. There was nothing special about the small menu. Everything on the menu was tofu cooked in various ways. I ordered some tofu and waited patiently for my food.

When I looked at the tofu on my plate I immediately noticed that the tofu looked shiny and smooth like a silky cloth. I had never seen such a good-looking tofu before. I hesitated for a moment before I put the first bite into my mouth. From the looks of this tofu, perhaps the cab driver knew what he was talking about! But the proof would be in the taste. I closed my eyes and concentrated on my first bite.

"Wonderful!" I shouted. "This is wonderful tofu!"

Do No Harm

I looked around the restaurant to see if anyone was looking at me and thinking I was crazy. I found myself yelling again with delight after my first mouthful of the most delicious taste I had ever experienced. I could not believe the silky texture and the deliciously smooth taste. I was actually making a spectacle of myself as I kept announcing to everyone how delighted I was to taste this wonderful dish!"

My waitress had come back to my table to make sure everything was all right.

"Excuse me, sir, is everything all right with your order?"

"Yes! Yes! This is the most delicious tofu I have ever tasted! I need to talk to the owner of the restaurant! Please tell him I would like to see him now!"

"Yes sir." The waitress looked a little bewildered, but left the room to find the owner. In a few moments a concerned-looking man approached my table.

"Yes, I am the owner of this restaurant. Is there a problem here? Are you displeased with your order?" he asked.

"No! No! There is not a problem with my food! I wanted to tell you that I have never had such a delicious tofu in all of my life! I have never seen such a beautiful texture, so silky and so smooth! Your tofu was recommended to me because it was the best, but I had no idea that your tofu would be this delicious! I am delighted with the taste and I wanted to ask you how you make this tofu so special. I know there are only a few ingredients in tofu and I'm trying to figure out what you do to make it so different from the tofu I have eaten before!"

I was obviously very excited and it was difficult for me to hold back my enthusiasm. The restaurant owner looked at me cautiously. He did not answer me immediately because he was looking me over and no doubt wondering if there was something wrong with me. I asked him if he could take a few minutes and sit down with me so I could explain to him who I was and why I was so interested in his tofu. Even though the restaurant was very busy, he kindly accepted my request and he sat down to listen.

After introducing myself and explaining why I was so curious about the tofu, he relaxed and asked me to calm down. He said, "Dr. Ohno, I see you are excited, but please calm down so I can answer your questions! It is the water, a very special water that has made this tofu so good. Tofu consists of 90% water; it is not a solid substance even though many people think of it as being solid. Because the water we use is a special water with very fine qualities, our tofu is exceptional to taste! This is not only true for tofu, but also for vegetables and fruits or even fish and meat. Anything that has water in it tastes better when the quality of the water is pure!"

"Both the ingredients and the water source for the tofu are from Japan. The soy is grown with this water to make the tofu. This is why this tofu is so delicious and different!"

My head was spinning with excitement and my heart was pounding as he talked about a special water that was so pure.

"Where do you purchase this water? Where does it come from? This is very important that I know!"

Again my excitement caused him to ask me to calm down. But I couldn't; I knew in my heart that I had been guided to this restaurant that day to find this water. I was fond of tofu, but never before had I wanted tofu so much that I would ask a cab driver to recommend a good tofu restaurant to me! It seemed as though I had been gently guided by some invisible force to have a craving for tofu that day so I would come here to learn about this special water. This would be too much of a coincidence for this water not to be the water I had been searching for. My excitement could not be contained.

"Dr. Ohno! Please, calm down! After you finish your meal, we can sit somewhere quietly and I can give you more information about where this water comes from!"

After I finished my tofu I joined him at a quiet area in the back. The waitress brought us both some tea and he proceeded to explain to me the history of this water.

"I discovered this water through my uncle. My uncle had been a cigarette smoker and he was suffering from lung cancer.

Do No Harm

When he was diagnosed with the lung cancer, the doctor said that the only alternative he could recommend was chemotherapy. So my uncle started with chemo treatments, but the side effects were so strong that he could not bear it. He finally asked his doctor to stop the chemotherapy. His doctor told him that if he stopped the treatments, he would have no chance of surviving. But my uncle was a stubborn man and he did not want to continue with the treatments any longer. So finally the doctor agreed to discharge my uncle from the hospital."

"After he left the hospital his symptoms became worse. He had to do something to help himself, so he turned to Oriental medicine. One day a friend advised him to visit a doctor who treated end-stage cancer patients. It seemed this doctor gave his patients a special water. After drinking the water for a period of time, their cancer would go into remission. His friend gave him the name of the doctor and told him the hospital where he was practicing."

"So, with nothing to lose, my uncle went to the hospital to find this doctor. Soon after meeting with the doctor, he was given this water. In a short time, his condition dramatically improved! His appetite, which had all but vanished, was back once again. My uncle was able to eat and started to gain weight. The tumors on his lung began to shrink, until eventually they were gone!"

"I know this is a difficult story to believe, but it is true! At first it was very difficult for me to believe that my uncle was cured from drinking water! If it had not been that this happened to my own uncle, who I know very well and witnessed his healing, I know I would not trust someone who would tell me such a far-fetched story. Six months after my uncle started drinking the water his lung cancer was in remission! Amazingly, Dr. Ohno, this is a true story."

"Tell me, Dr. Ohno, what do you think about this story?"

I told him that I believed what he told me was possible and I trusted that this water could have special properties that aided in the healing of his uncle's cancer. He was happy to see that I

Yoshitaka Ohno, M.D., Ph.D.

believed his story. He went on to say, "I have tried to explain this story to many of my friends, and even though they know me very well, they find it difficult to believe me. In order to further prove this to myself, I decided to drink this water, because I had hypertension and diabetes. I thought that if the water could help my uncle with lung cancer, perhaps it could help with my health problems as well. Every day, I had to take medication for my high blood pressure, and insulin for my diabetes. Shortly after I started to drink this magnetized water, my blood pressure dropped from 180/120 to 120/78! My glucose level dropped from 300 to where it is now at 120! I will always drink a bottle of this water every day to maintain my health."

"I have also discovered that I experience more energy than I did before! It used to be difficult for me to get up in the morning because I was always so tired. Now, even if I go to bed after midnight, I wake up in the morning between 5-6 AM feeling refreshed.

After taking a break and sipping some more tea, the restaurant owner continued with his story.

"After my uncle and I had such a good experience with this water, I thought of the idea of using this water for cooking in my restaurant. I knew that because tofu was made up of 90% water, that the purity of the water would make a big difference in the taste and the quality of the tofu. So, I started using the water in my restaurant and I never said anything to anyone about it. But within a short period of time, I had a great increase in business. People from all over have come to taste our tofu!"

His story intrigued me and I wanted to learn more about the water. I also wanted to meet the doctor who was administering the water to his cancer patients. I asked him, "Where can I go to meet this doctor and find out more about this special water?"

"The doctor you want to talk to is at Shibata Hospital in Okayama. His name is Dr. Jinro Itami. I can give you directions how to get there."

Do No Harm

Dr. Itami, Shibata Hospital
Okayama, Japan

After I returned home, I scheduled an appointment to see Dr. Itami. I made the three-hour trip from Osaka to Okayama and the Shibata Hospital. Even though the hospital looked humble and small, I felt a special energy from the building and from the staff when I walked inside. I waited for 10 minutes and Dr. Itami, a man about 50 years old, came over and introduced himself. His voice was soft and caring, and his eyes were kind and compassionate. I felt immediately that I could trust him. And this proved to be true. He was generous with his time during that first visit, as he took time out of his busy schedule from seeing his patients.

"Welcome, Dr. Ohno! Welcome to Shibata Hospital! I am so glad to meet you! I have been looking forward to meeting you, especially after our conversation about the water over the phone. There aren't many doctors who understand the importance of water and how it affects our body!"

I was impressed with Dr. Itami and his humility from our first conversation. When he discussed his patients and how they have been healed, he never indicated to me that he was taking the credit. He always gave the credit to the water. He had said, "I am not curing the patients, it is the water that is making the difference. I am only giving them the water."

Now that I had met him in person, I was able to confirm that he was indeed a sweet and modest man. His attitude was very different from the typical Japanese doctors I was used to associating with, who were generally arrogant. The more I talked with him, the more I liked him. He was a true humanitarian and meeting him inspired me. I was now even more excited about discussing the water with him.

"Please tell me about this special water, Dr. Itami. How long have you been using it with your patients?"

"I have been using the water with end-stage cancer patients now for 10 years, Dr. Ohno. I have kept records since I started giving it to my cancer patients!"

"What can you tell me about your findings?"

"Most of the patients visit me at this hospital after they have moved into the end stages of cancer. Most of these patients have already gone through radiation, surgery, chemotherapy, and immunotherapy. Many patients have been to several doctors, who offered them new 'cures' for cancer. Most of these patients have lost trust in their doctors because none of them seemed to improve. Their hopes have been dimmed, and they are scared of facing death. They are looking for a miracle that can give them hope and a chance to live. Even though I do not claim to work miracles, I believe I have given many of my patients hope in helping them to deal with their cancer. You see, Dr. Ohno, my mission in medicine is to give people hope. Even if I am not able to cure them of their cancer, at least I want to give them hope."

"Years ago I heard about a mountain that was being mined. The miners who worked there drank the water that came out of the mountain. Many of these miners were suffering from health problems; such as arthritis, hypertension, diabetes, kidney stones, to name a few. After drinking this water over a period of time, they discovered that their health improved and some of their symptoms had disappeared altogether. When I heard about this from some of the miners, I began to wonder if there would be benefits from this water for my cancer patients. Even though I was skeptical, I decided it was at least worth trying."

"I knew that my patients would try anything to cure their cancer. You know the saying: *A drowning man will reach for a straw.* In other words, a dying man will try anything that will help him live.

Dr. Itami invited me to take a stroll with him to visit some of his patients. One of the first patients Dr. Itami pointed out was a young man, 42 years old. He had just been admitted into the hospital with liver cancer. Dr. Itami told me, "This man was told

Do No Harm

that he has only three months to live. He is in the end-stages of liver cancer and the cancer has metastasized to his major organs. His doctor told him that there was nothing they could do to help him, and he should go to hospice. His wife had heard from a friend about our work here and how the water was helping to cure cancer in some patients."

I looked at the man with his belly swollen like a sumo wrestler. He was dreadfully thin and he looked very tired. I reached out my hand to shake his as I introduced myself. I asked him, "How are you feeling?"

The patient said, "I have had no appetite even though my abdomen is growing larger from the swelling ever day. But I have not given up because many of my friends have told me about Dr. Itami and his special water. I am hoping that this water will cure my liver cancer. This is my last chance. I know I can trust you, Dr. Itami, because I have been told that you are a true caring and compassionate person. I believe that you can help me!"

Dr. Itami listened and looked down, smiling shyly. As we walked away, he explained to me, "I will start giving the water to him right away. I hope that the water will give him new hope. But all I can do is my best and allow the water to work in his body. The rest is up to God."

As we continued to walk through the hospital ward, many patients smiled and waved to Dr. Itami. One patient in particular called him over, "Dr. Itami! Thank you so much for helping me! You have given me so much hope. I have never had another doctor care for me in the way you do. I am so thankful that I came here so you could help me. Even though I may die here, Dr. Itami, I will never regret it because I found a doctor I could trust!"

I watched Dr. Itami as many patients sang his praises. Never once did he show an attitude of conceit. He smiled to every patient, and he made everyone feel at ease. I witnessed his humanitarian behavior. He was really a special and unusual doctor. He was not caught up in ego and greed. Rather, he was fueled by his mission to give hope to patients, who had nothing left to turn to but hope and prayer.

Something I felt was amazing with these patients. I could understand how the woman who had been here for awhile talked about trusting Dr. Itami. But the liver cancer patient who had just been admitted to the hospital already trusted Dr. Itami. I wondered how it was that he was able to gain the trust of this patient so quickly, even before giving the patient any kind of care.

I remembered when my mother had her breast cancer operation. I recalled how she told me that she trusted my brother Yoshioki because there was a special spiritual energy that worked between them. I believed in this energy and knew that it was imperative for the healing process to be successful.

"Dr. Itami, how do you go about gaining the complete trust of your patients? You seem to have a gift for gaining a patient's trust. How are you able to do this?"

"Dr. Ohno, when my patients come here, I am often times their very last hope. Usually they have already seen several doctors and have gone through taking several different kinds of drugs and therapies. Nothing has worked for them or they would not be here. Most of these patients have lost their trust in doctors and the medical profession. They see their lives slipping helplessly away. When they first are admitted to the hospital, they do not know that I am any different from other doctors. Because they need to gain hope and trust before they can begin to get better, I help them by the way I treat them."

"The first thing I do is ask the patient to relax. I acknowledge that I know they are scared and I talk with them in a caring way. I spend the first three days getting to know them as a person. I ask them questions about their life, their family, what they do for a living, or I ask them to share with me what they want me to know about them. It's not until after the third day that I begin to discuss their medical history with them. By the time I begin to treat them medically, we have developed a relationship that is based upon the deepest human factors of trust and faith. I continue to remind them to relax and I always listen to their fears and concerns. Quickly, I am able to give the patient hope and in return, they are able to give me their trust. Both must work together, Dr. Ohno, for healing to occur."

From everything I was experiencing from talking with him and watching him with his patients, I truly liked and respected Dr. Itami. He was everything I felt he was from my first impression. He was kind and compassionate; a true humanitarian doctor. I was very impressed with him. When we returned to his office, I asked him, "Dr. Itami, what is it about this water that makes it so special?"

"I'm not sure why the water works on diseases, but I do know the history of this water. Almost a billion years ago, there was an undersea volcano that erupted in this area. When the volcano erupted it rose up out of the ocean and became a mountain. Following the volcano eruption there was a huge meteorite shower in this same area. The magnetite in the meteorites bonded with the limestone and granite of the mountain. This created a permanent magnetic mountain.

"As water flows into the mountain, it is magnetized with the mountain's magnetic field. Because of its magnetism, the water is able to attract 74 minerals that are in the mountain. Some of these minerals are calcium, magnesium, selenium, and potassium, gold, silver, iron. What is equally important about this mineral water is the ionic organization of its structure. The mineral water has an organized ionization that is unique. When this water is inside our bodies, it helps to create a healthy environment." I was in complete agreement with Dr. Itami because he confirmed everything I knew about water and magnetism.

Dr. Itami asked me to join him for lunch near the hospital. There was a restaurant that was famous for its vegetable menu. When we entered the restaurant I saw a small pond filled with fish. I looked at this pond and I tried to figure out what kind of fish were in there. At first I thought they might be salmon. But Dr. Itami told me that they were not salmon, they were trout. I couldn't believe they were trout because they were so large! The size of the trout was nearly double normal size. Dr. Itami explained that these trout were swimming in the same water that he gave to his patients.

The food in the restaurant was delicious! Everything from the tea, to the vegetables, to the fish! The food melted in my mouth and I knew that all of this food must be good for my body as well. I asked Dr. Itami, "How are you able to get this water from the source of the mountain?"

"I go to the mountain twice a week to get the water. Since the water is so heavy, the shipping cost is expensive. It takes about an hour to get to the mountain from here, but it is worth the drive. After I get the water, I give it to my patients."

Dr. Itami continued to amaze me. He traveled one hour each way to get the water from the mountain twice a week, to get this water to his patients. This further confirmed what a special person he is. Dr. Itami explained to me how to find Nariwa Village, where the mountain is located. There, right at the mountain is a bottling company that takes the water from the mountain before the water can be contaminated by the environment. He told me to go to the bottling company and ask for the owner. This man would be able to answer any questions I had regarding the water.

As we started to leave I hoped that when I got to Nariwa Village, I would find what I had been searching for. This could be the moment when my life would shift and my world would never be the same again. I expressed my gratitude and appreciation as I said good-bye to Dr. Itami.

Nariwa Village
Home of the Source

*Invisible energy guides your life through intuition
Learning not to question but to acknowledge your instincts
Leads you to your rightful place*

The countryside leading to Nariwa Village from Okayama is one of the most scenic areas of Japan. There are rolling hills with plush landscape, and the rich vegetation is everywhere. The air is sweet from the fresh smell of the evergreens. The winding road led me deeper and deeper into the interior of the countryside, and the foothills gave way to a cascade of mountains. The mountains were green and beautiful, yet not overwhelming. I felt strangely at home here. I felt as though I were simply returning to a place I had visited before. As I came closer to the area where the magnetic mountain was, I could feel an adrenaline rush in my body. It was a magical moment in time for me, as I knew I was coming closer and closer to the source of the water.

High upon a winding mountain road was the bottling company Dr. Itami told me about. I went in and asked to see the owner. A kind gentleman with a broad smile and a hearty handshake came out and introduced himself to me as Mr. Hanaoka. I told him who I was and why I had come. He graciously asked if I would like to see the water in the mountain. After giving me a tour from the top of the mountain, I asked him to tell me everything he could about the mountain and the water.

"This water comes from the ceiling inside the mountain, as well as from an underground pool."

"How much water can be taken from the mountain?" I asked.

"The water source is huge. I suppose you could get around 200,000 gallons of water a day. But our bottling facility does not have capacity to bottle that much. Currently, we are only getting

Yoshitaka Ohno, M.D., Ph.D.

the water from one small branch coming off the main source. When there is a greater demand for this water, I'm sure we could bottle much more.

"If this water is so special, why is it not well known, I asked?"

"There are over 300 different bottled water companies in Japan. With so many water companies, it is hard for people to distinguish the differences between these waters. Many people think that all water is the same, but I'm sure you know that this is not true."

"That's right," I said. "Unless people are educated to know the difference in the quality of water, they cannot determine which water is best for their health!

This water is the best I have ever heard of, not only in Japan, but also worldwide!

Then Mr. Hanaoka continued, "As far as I know, our water is the only naturally magnetized water that has been found! It would take another miraculous act of nature like what happened here in order for this phenomenon to be created again!"

After seeing the mountain and visiting with Mr. Hanaoka, I was now even more inspired by what I had heard about the minerals and magnetic properties of this naturally magnetized water. From my studies of geology, magnetism, astronomy and water, I believed that there could definitely be something special about this water that made it different from any other water source. Because I was inspired by Dr. Itami's work with his cancer patients, I was eager to get back to my research with this water to develop my theory, that magnetized water could have an effect on improving human health.

I believe that this water could improve symptoms of Alzheimer's patients. After meeting Dr. Itami, I understood why this water could help improve patients with cancer and other diseases. Years ago before my father died, one of his dreams had been to establish an institute for research purposes. I believed that the energy of his thoughts had transferred to me, and I was destined to start the Ohno Institute for Research. My father's dream became my dream. But my dream would also allow me to research the benefits of the naturally magnetized water for health.

Fulfilling A Legacy

*We are meant to do what brings us joy in life.
That is why we are given certain gifts and
interests for specific areas.
The areas we feel a true passion are the
areas we are meant to pursue.*

So it was that I established the Ohno Institute in Osaka, as a part of the Ohno Hospital. I had published a book on treating Alzheimer's patients that attracted attention in Japan. Because of my book, people contacted me to learn more about this disease. Most of the people who contacted me had family members with Alzheimer's. I used this opportunity to introduce the naturally magnetized water I had discovered to them, and began research on the water and its effects on Alzheimer's patients. I also received referrals for my studies from the Ohno Hospital. For the people in my studies who had lost hope, I believed I could at least offer them that. I had faith in the healing properties of this water, which gave me an even stronger faith in my purpose in life.

One of the subjects in my study was a friend of mine who was a dialysis patient. He had suffered from diabetes, which ultimately led to kidney deficiency. He had been on dialysis twice a week for over 10 years. He was put on water restriction and told to limit drinking water to one liter a day. He was a big water drinker and told me he was always thirsty. From time to time he would question me about my research and the special magnetized water he knew I was studying.

"I would like to try your water!"

Yoshitaka Ohno, M.D., Ph.D.

"I don't want to get in trouble with your doctor," I said. "Water has too many chemicals and is dangerous to dialysis patients. I don't think your doctor would understand that my water is different and could help you."

Finally, one day he said to me, "Look, my friend, before I die from kidney failure, I would like to drink your water! I don't care what my doctor says."

"I have never tried the water with a dialysis patient," I said, "and I am not comfortable giving it to you because of your required water restriction."

"Dr. Ohno, then I will be your first dialysis patient to drink this water! If you want me to sign a paper relieving you of responsibility, I will gladly do that! I have lost my job, my wife has divorced me, and I have nothing left in my life. All I request before I die is to drink your water!"

I rejected his proposal until I heard from a mutual friend that he had attempted to commit suicide. Fortunately, he had failed in his attempt, but since he was so determined I decided to give him some of the water. I went to the hospital to visit him and said, "O.K., I am going to give you some water, but you must understand that we are going to begin with very small amounts! If you see that you are experiencing a bad reaction from drinking this water, then you must tell me immediately so we can stop! This is something we need to agree on!"

"Yes! Thank you! I will do my best to cooperate with you!"

In the beginning I gave him only a half glass of water. He was disappointed that it wasn't more, but I wanted to see if he would have any reaction to the water.

"Tomorrow", I said, "we will try the same amount. Before I see you tomorrow, I want to make sure you are all right. If this water causes you to have any reactions, then I will have to stop giving it to you!"

The next day I gave him a small amount of water and we monitored him closely. He was doing fine so I increased the amount. After one week he was drinking eight ounces a day. By the end of one month he was up to 16 ounces. His kidney

Do No Harm

function began to improve. He also began to have more frequent urination. I told him he should keep drinking 16 ounces of this water every day. He continued to improve, and one year later he was completely off dialysis!

I remember finally telling his doctor about giving him my water. The doctor said, "Dr. Ohno, if you weren't a doctor, I would be very upset. I didn't know why he improved and could get off dialysis. I thought it was just one of those mysteries we see often in medicine. But maybe your water has got something special."

Then I said something I thought was important. "If my water can allow a dialysis patient to drink my water and not decrease kidney function or create edema, shouldn't we try it with all of your dialysis patients? Shouldn't this water be a part of their treatment protocol?"

He looked at me as if I had just suggested using voodoo as a treatment. He just turned away and ignored me.

I gave him a report from one of my studies and offered to give him some of the water. Just as I suspected, he refused, saying that there is really no way water could make a difference. This was typical of the responses I had been getting from doctors since I found this water. I walked away thinking that maybe medicine wasn't ready to accept this water. After all, it didn't come from a pharmaceutical company.

The Ohno Institute was getting very good results from the patients we tested with this water. I was finding the research very rewarding because I was once again giving hope to many patients who needed it desperately. I continued my contact with Dr. Itami and discussed with him the idea of publishing our results together in a medical journal. I anticipated that he would be excited, but I was wrong.

"Dr.Ohno, my honest opinion is that it is not a good idea to publish our results! I know how excited you are about the research you've been conducting over the past year, and I know you are encouraged by the potential this water has to help many more people. But please keep in mind the Japanese Medical

Yoshitaka Ohno, M.D., Ph.D.

Society will fight to have your ideas rejected. The pharmaceutical companies control them, and they are not going to want to publish our results, no matter how positive they may be! I had attempted to publish my findings before, but they said my research was fake and that I was receiving money from the water company as compensation!"

"Dr. Ohno, you are a good doctor. I like your work ethic and I have seen that you are a true humanitarian, wanting to bring hope to people's lives. I know you have the potential to help many people, not just Japanese, but people from all over the world! You will be a hero to many people some day. People here need you, but I don't think you can do what you want to do in Japan. I think you will need to go back to America where they are more acceptant of your ideas! If you attempt to publish your results in Japan, they will laugh at you and say that you are just trying to make a name for yourself."

"Even though I have collected data from my patients who have benefited from the naturally magnetized water and reported my findings, I do not have any influence with our medical society. My hospital is small and it is not recognized by the medical society as a valid research facility. If this were a large school such as Tokyo Medical University, then I would have a much better opportunity to get my findings published. You are well aware of the politics here, and how difficult it is for doctors such as you and me to break through years of conservative thinking."

"I have gone through many years of criticism and ridicule from other doctors. They say that I have never really healed anyone with this water. They have called me a liar and have accused me of all sorts of things. But I know I am not a liar."

All of a sudden Dr. Itami had tears in his eyes. I realized that he and I had something in common. Both of us had been criticized and scorned by our peers for our untraditional thinking and willingness to risk our reputations. Both of us were not part of the Japanese Medical Society's politics. We were doctors

Do No Harm

who needed to give hope to their patients by using whatever methods possible. We were allies of the heart.

I knew what he told me was true. I had actually known this to be true right along. I had just hoped that after the results we both had gotten from our studies, that together we could overcome the system and publish our findings.

Perhaps he was right. Maybe I needed to return once again to America. I had proven to myself before what I could accomplish on my own, when I made my mind up to do something important. Maybe I needed to go to America to establish the Ohno Institute for research. I was beginning to understand that life was always going to be challenging, and I needed to go where I was guided to go.

Yoshitaka Ohno, M.D., Ph.D.

Chapter Eight

Bringing Japan's Gift of Life to America

Sometimes when a gift is freely given, it is rejected as Valueless because it is Free

When I returned to Osaka, I spent much of my time at the Ohno Institute contacting people whom I had met in Denver. I asked them to recommend universities or institutes where research on Alzheimer's disease was being conducted. Responses were very slow and I became discouraged. I contacted these facilities and requested help in pursuing my research on the naturally magnetized water, but no one was even slightly interested. In fact, I could tell by the tone of their voices that they thought I was just another "new age" scientist who knew nothing about scientific investigation.

One day we had a visitor from America come to Osaka to lecture on Alzheimer's care. I was in the audience, and after the lecture, I introduced myself to him. He was the president of a hospital near Cleveland, Ohio called Heather Hill. Through my work in Alzheimer's research, I had read about this facility. I had heard that Heather Hill was a very good specialty hospital and health care facility that gave exceptional care for Alzheimer's patients. He seemed to be very receptive to my ideas and my interest in coming to America to pursue my research on the relationship between water and disease. By the end of our talk, he asked me to consider coming to his facility to do my research.

About three weeks later, I contacted the president at Heather Hill, and after discussing my work in Japan with Alzheimer's patients, he offered me a position as Research Fellow to do studies on my water. It seemed like the opportunity I was

Do No Harm

waiting for, so I decided to move from Osaka, Japan to Cleveland, Ohio, U.S.A.

I remember the conditions given to me by the president regarding my position. Instead of receiving a salary, I was asked to make a large donation to his hospital to cover the expenses of my research. I thought that this was unusual, but I was so anxious to get to America to continue my research that I decided to accept the terms of his offer.

I discussed this with my mother. She knew immediately that I might have been taken advantage of, but she felt that this "investment" in my future was worth it. Instead of alerting me to the disappointment I might find there, she gave me her blessing and said that she would have the president of Heather Hill contacted to make the arrangements. I have found over the years that my passion for my work has sometimes led me blindly to accept being exploited.

In spite of my mother's concern and wise counseling, I was excited about doing clinical studies on the effect of the naturally magnetized water on cognitive function with the Alzheimer's patients at Heather Hill. My ultimate goal was to publish my findings in an American medical journal. I hoped that publishing my research would draw interest and give me credibility in the American medical community regarding my ideas about water and why the quality of water is so vital to our health.

But several months of patiently waiting to begin my study turned into three long and frustrating years! After receiving several promises from the research director and the president of the hospital, it became clear that I was never going to get the help I needed. After substantial donations from my family and unsuccessfully negotiating with them to start my study, one of the reasons I was given was the fact that Heather Hill was not a university, but a health care facility, meaning my study would be difficult to publish.

Later on, the research director would honestly tell me, "I had to reject your proposal for a study because I was afraid of the political problems it would cause, and I did not want to jeopardize my position at Heather Hill."

After the director repeatedly came up with reasons as to why I could not do research, I visited several universities in the surrounding area. I talked to many medical professors and many physicians about the naturally magnetized water and asked if they would help me with a clinical study, or help me secure a grant for my research. Everywhere I went I was turned down and sometimes I was even laughed at. There was no one I met that I could persuade to listen to my ideas or look at my data. Unfortunately, I found the American medical establishment as political as the Japan Medical Society.

I kept thinking there was something I was doing wrong. I believed in the special healing power of this water, but every one I talked to turned my ideas down. I had hoped that by coming to America I would connect with more people who were open minded and had the spirit of accepting new ideas that America was founded on.

During the three years after returning to America, I couldn't find anyone to listen to my theory about water and all the work I had done. After being in America for awhile, I noticed that there were very few books about water and health. Even in Japan there were many books in bookstores about water. Perhaps it is because water in Japan is such a precious commodity that there is much more awareness of water and the environment. In America there seems to be little interest about the importance of clean water in our bodies. It is no wonder that people continue to get sick and don't know why. Even when people are aware of the dangers of water contamination, they don't know about the effect water has on the human body.

We think of the body consisting of muscles, bones and nerves. But everything in our body is made up of almost all water. Our body is made up of 70% water. Too much of our health education is about drugs and the effects certain drugs have on the body. How often do we hear about water and its effects on our health? All of the foods we eat consist of water. Good water produces good crops that keep us healthy. When we eat vegetables that have been grown in a contaminated field from chemicals and polluted soil, we are not providing our body with nourishment, but poison. When we eat poultry, beef, pork or fish that has been contaminated from a poor water source, are we not poisoned as well?

The awareness in America is slowly growing. Since so little is taught about the importance of water in the body, it is easy for people to contaminate their bodies without being aware of what they are doing. Since we are the unity of a mind/body/spirit relationship, it makes sense that not only is our body contaminated by poor water, but our mind and our spirit as well. When we do not take proper care of our body, the body cannot remain in a balanced state. Water helps to balance our body, and when we are balanced physically, our emotions are much more stable. We become less irritable and angry, and our spiritual energy is much more alive.

"Danger Past, God Forgotten"

It is amazing to me that it usually takes a crisis for people to wake up and understand how vital water is. Most people ignore how important our water resources are until they experience a problem. The earth is also made up of 70% water. But 94% of our water supply is salt water. Only 6% of our earth's water is fresh water. Of this 4% is in the form of glaciers. This leaves approximately 2% fresh water on earth for human consumption. If we continue to ignore water as the very precious commodity it is, we are in danger of destroying not just our bodies; we are in danger of also destroying our home planet, Earth.

Many people have called me the "Water Doctor," saying that all I know is water. All I want to talk about is water. I try to be understanding, but without knowledge about the importance of water, my words sound too simplistic to have any merit.

I had gotten used to people laughing at me and telling me that my ideas are not reality. I am used to the feeling of alienation and exclusion, so attempts to discourage me have not affected my determination. I continue to focus on the benefits of the water I discovered, and I tell people about this water anytime I have the opportunity to do so. Usually, when I meet someone with a health problem, or they tell me about someone in their family with a health problem, they say they have tried every kind of conventional medical treatment available. But after seeing no improvements, they have lost hope. I am always eager to help them. I will explain the special qualities of the water, and how the water I discovered in Japan can help them. When I get this opportunity, people will listen to me.

One day a woman visited Heather Hill because she was looking for a good facility to care for her sister who had Alzheimer's disease. She toured the facility but was terribly disappointed when she realized she would not be able to afford the cost of care. I was very impressed with her devotion to her sister, and I took a few minutes to talk to her about her sister's state of health.

"Excuse me, my name is Dr. Ohno. I understand that your sister is suffering from Alzheimer's disease. I suppose that even though you have tried to do a good job in taking care of her at home, her symptoms are getting worse. I can see that you look very tired from the strain of taking care of her. I would like to tell you about something that can help your sister. It is naturally magnetized water. I have had good results giving this water to Alzheimer's patients." I explained to her.

"I came to Heather Hill to do studies with this water. I have used it in studies in Japan and the results with Alzheimer's patients have been very encouraging. If you are truly interested in trying this water on your sister, I will be happy to help you!"

"Dr. Ohno, I have tried everything I can think of! I cannot afford to bring my sister to Heather Hill and I cannot take care of her by myself anymore. Let me try your water and see if at least this helps her. Any improvement to her health will be appreciated!"

Do No Harm

I delivered a case of the water to her home the next day. I instructed her to have her sister drink one bottle of water each day and to record any differences she saw in her sister's behavior.

After one month, she reported that her sister's cognitive functioning had improved. Her eyes no longer looked dull, but sharp and alert. Her appetite had improved dramatically and she was able to walk much better. After two months of drinking the water daily, she again began to distinguish people and recognize who they were!

"Who am I?" she asked when she and her sister visited me.

"You are my sister!" she answered.

"Dr. Ohno! I cannot tell you what it means to me to have my sister recognize me again! I have to tell you, I was really skeptical before trying your water. I am so glad you approached me and told me about this water! I need you to explain what is happening to my sister and why this water is able to help her."

"I am so happy that your sister is improving so nicely! Thank you very much for asking this question! It has not been often since I came to Heather Hill that someone has wanted me to explain to them about this water. I believe that this water can help people with any disease, not just Alzheimer's!

I answered her as simply as I could.

"There are 100 billion cells in the brain, and the brain is made up of 90% water. One of the reasons Alzheimer's disease occurs is because of contamination of the water which composes the brain. When the brain cells become contaminated, they lose electrons. The brain cells then cease to function and they cannot send the information correctly. This happens because the contaminated cells become disorganized and unstable. So the signals that normally create impulses that travel from one cell to another are no longer in a stable environment and are unable to transfer information correctly. My theory is that if we can improve the water in the brain, we can improve the responses of the brain.

Yoshitaka Ohno, M.D., Ph.D.

The reason why naturally magnetized water helps to improve cognitive functioning, like memory, is because the water is highly organized. Once this water enters the cells of the brain, the cells become organized and the impulses once again connect. Keep in mind this is a very simplistic explanation, but it helps to give you an idea as to why the water is helping your sister."

She was very surprised to hear my explanation. "I would never have believed your theory until I saw the results! I am a chemist and I can see where the quality of the water would definitely impact the functioning. I just have never really thought it would affect it to that extent!"

"If you were not a chemist than perhaps you would not have understood my idea, I responded."

"Dr. Ohno, if you have so much trouble getting studies done at Heather Hill and they do not appreciate what this wonderful water could do for their patients, why don't you open up your own clinic? Just think of the people you could help!"

I was so appreciative of her suggestion. I had met very few people who were as kind and understanding as she was. The compassion she had given to her sister, and the concern she was extending to me was heartfelt. I left her home that day feeling as though I was the one who had been healed. I decided to give strong consideration to her idea. I had, after all, opened the Ohno Institute before in Osaka and my work had been very rewarding. Her suggestion made a lot of sense to me and was something I would definitely think about.

> *"Life consists of destiny.*
> *Whether you experience good destiny or not,*
> *depends upon your effort ~*
> *The Destiny that comes into your life is not an accident"*

Meeting this woman and helping her sister was very important for me. I felt the timing was perfect. My hope was

Do No Harm

diminishing and I had started to consider moving back to Japan. But as with so many events in my life, something always seems to happen at the right moment to put my life back in order. I felt this was a sign for me to try to continue my journey in finding support for my projects. What I needed was to find someone who had the knowledge to understand my ideas, and the ability to help me get started. I knew this was going to happen soon.

In 1995 it began to happen. The director of research at Heather Hill was replaced by Dr. Howard Reminick. I was told of Dr. Reminick, and anticipated his arrival. All I could hope was that this wouldn't be another administrator whose ego and political ambitions were more important than his willingness to help.

Dr. Reminick had a Ph.D. in medical research and education, with a very good reputation. I was anxious to meet with him and to see if he would be open and receptive in his thinking to the idea of using the naturally magnetized water in a study at Heather Hill. Upon meeting with Dr. Reminick, I was immediately impressed by his generous smile and warmth. I couldn't believe his willingness to listen to me, even before he got settled in his office. I had a very good feeling about this man, and felt he would be someone with whom I could share my ideas. I invited him to lunch so we could get to know each other better.

I shared my background with him and my unconventional ideas about the naturally magnetized water. I told him about my studies in Japan and why I had not stayed there to pursue my research. I also told him how disappointed I had been for the past three years, because I could not get anyone here to support me. I told him about the broken promises made to me by the previous research director and my frustration over missing opportunities to help people. I also told him how I was helping patients secretly, and that I had documented my findings on how this water had improved health.

It was difficult for Dr. Reminick to understand my theory of magnetized water because he had never heard of magnetized water before. But fortunately, he understood magnetic fields and magnetism in the body. He had worked on the development of TENS and Functional Electrical Stimulators. He also had previous experience researching water-filtering processes, and he knew a great deal about water. He had been a professor of health education and had his research studies published. He knew the dangers of our drinking water and how it affects health.

Even though Dr.Reminick admitted to not being an expert, I was excited to see that he had a genuine interest in what I was doing and, he showed a willingness to learn more about it. Most important, he suggested that we begin to design a study right away!

Dr. Howard Reminick soon became "Howard" to me. Howard quickly became my associate, my ally and my friend. As our relationship grew and I saw him make things happen, I was sure that I was home in America to stay.

An Oasis in the Desert

"Friends are our chosen family"

In addition to helping me design and write the proposal for my study, Howard was able to discuss my work and the theory of the water intelligently with the Heather Hill staff. Even those who were skeptical and ridiculed my ideas were now listening with interest. Howard brought my ideas into the larger medical community, promoting my work by doing lectures and conferences throughout the country. He was able to gain the curiosity of many professionals. All of a sudden I was being sought out as someone scientifically knowledgeable who had an idea worth researching and developing. Howard became my communicator and promoter. As he learned more about water, magnetism and health, he was able to speak and write about the benefits of the naturally magnetized water.

Our Alzheimer's study at Heather Hill was completed. When we analyzed the data, we found significant differences in memory retention between the subjects in the experimental group, who were given the naturally magnetized water for six months, and the subjects in the control group, who drank only tap water. Since we found significant results from the study, we were hopeful to have our findings published. But our hopes were crushed when the article we submitted to many journals was rejected. We were told, "Sorry. This is not a good study because the sample was not large enough. We told the journals that this subject was never studied before; and this study was a pilot so we could determine if it was feasible to do a larger study.

There were thousands of dollars of my money invested in this study. Both Howard and I were bewildered as what to do to get our findings published. Finally, a journal, *Frontier Perspectives, the Journal of Frontier Sciences of Temple University,* accepted our paper and it was published in the fall of 1997. We knew that we wanted to do further studies with the water and other diseases, such as cancer, arthritis, multiple sclerosis and more. Whenever someone contacted us and requested the water, we asked them to keep a record on their reactions and improvements, so we could report the results. We soon recognized that we needed to establish our own research organization. So in June of 1998, we opened the Ohno Institute on Water and Health, a non-profit organization.

At that time I brought in a new associate, Ken Haibara, to help us with our work. Ken had a background in technology. He assisted with managing the administrative functions of the Institute.

Our work progressed slowly as we made connections with doctors to set up study sites. We sent the water to them for their patients and asked that data be kept and a report sent after the study. Even though it has been a struggle to finance our Institute, the people who have benefited from this water with significant improvement to their health have made it worthwhile.

Yoshitaka Ohno, M.D., Ph.D.

Expanding Our Mission from the Clinic to the World

The Japanese Festival of Mind/Body/Spirit Health at the Smithsonian Institute

*The only component that separates us from each other
Is not the color of our skin or the home of our ancestry,
The only component that separates us from each other
Lies within the degree of openness in our heart.*

My uncle, Dr. Yoriaki Hamuro, the Chief Priest at Kasuga Taisha shrine in Nara, Japan came to America in September 1999, for a special Japanese Festival I hosted at the Smithsonian in Washington D.C. A year earlier I had hosted a successful Japanese Festival at the Cleveland Art Museum that featured Taiko Drumming, a synchronized Japanese drumming art form. This was the most attended event of its kind ever held there, and it was on Labor Day weekend! The theme of both festivals was Harmony Between Mankind and Nature. I wanted to emphasize our dependency on the forces and spirit of Nature, and the gratitude we should be constantly expressing. I also presented what I believe to be Nature's most precious gift, the water we drink to live. The traditions of Shinto, unique to Japan, are founded on this philosophy.

There were 15 members of the Japanese party that accompanied my uncle, including my mother. My uncle had been delighted when I extended him the invitation to come to America and speak to an American audience. His special message that he had been delivering to the Japanese people was becoming popular, and he was getting requests to travel to several countries to speak. Most audiences expected a Chief

Do No Harm

Priest to talk about religion, but Dr. Hamuro surprised everyone by talking about the relationship of man, nature and water.

In the Shinto philosophy the element of honoring and feeling gratitude to nature is the main message which expresses the beliefs of the Japanese culture. But as with all modern day cultures, the importance of the Shinto philosophy is slowly disappearing into the stressful lifestyle of modern Japan. Japan has been trying to keep up with American life style, and the younger generation has lost much of the ancestral values, such as gratitude for living in harmony with nature that was so vital in past decades.

As soon as Dr. Hamuro began to speak, all eyes were locked on him as he inspired the large audience. I realized that he was reinforcing what I was doing to practice his humanitarian message. After the festival was over, we discussed how the Shinto philosophy stressed the importance of preserving the quality of water for our future generations. I shared with my mother and my uncle the difficulty I was having in getting people to become more receptive to learning about the special water I had brought from Japan.

I struggled to come up with a name that would express what I believed and what I had learned from my many years of study and research on health and aging. I needed a name that would be synonymous with the concept of giving hope to people who longed for inner peace and good health, and understood that what we do to our earth we do to ourselves. The name that came to me was Shintopia, a combination of Shinto and Utopia. It was then that I received a clearer view of what I wanted to achieve in my search to become a better person. I will discuss my vision of Shintopia in the next chapter

Someday, when people are more receptive to what I have to say and realize that I truly want to help them, I would like to build a Mind/Body/Spirit Healing Retreat Center, where people could come to learn and practice how to be in harmony with nature. This will be a place where they can renew their spirit and learn to use nature's gifts, such as its best water. Someday perhaps I will be able to see this dream come true. I want this to be a place where people gain a new awareness that they can hold in their heart, in their mind, and in their soul.

There is no limit to the healing that can take place ~
When appreciation is applied to your consciousness.

I know that the challenges I have experienced have helped me to become a more compassionate and humanitarian person. I also know that I have been guided by a divine spiritual energy to find the special, naturally magnetized water that has brought hope to so many people. After years of watching how people's lives have been changed by drinking this water, I am a firm believer of its power and will always continue to share it with every one I can.

Even though I have studied many branches of science and medicine, what has affected me the most has been the metaphysical principles I have learned. Of these principles, the strong interrelationship of mind/body/spirit continues to intrigue me the more I learn to use it. As much as I believe in the healing power of the naturally magnetized water, I am convinced that this water will only help a person to the degree their belief system will allow. This is true with anything in our life. The more we can understand the nature of cause and effect and how our actions create the threads that interconnect our mind/body/spirit nature, the more power we can possess within to take total command of Self.

Through my years of involvement in the medical field, working directly with patients who are very ill, and through all of my experience in research, looking for answers to disease and aging, I have made many discoveries as to the *potential* that the individual possesses for healing. The ability of people to heal themselves is much more than finding a good doctor or using the

Do No Harm

best drugs, or even drinking the special water that I have come to believe in.

I have used the phrase "invisible energy." I believe that there is a union of energy that transfers between the doctor and the patient. It is vital that there be a bond of trust and compassion between them. The patients must be able to trust the physician in order for their bodies to respond positively for healing. And the doctors must feel compassion for their patients before anything they do will have effective results. Without this energy transference between doctor and patient, a return to health is not going to be successful.

Beyond the patient – doctor relationship, there is yet another vital component that must be present before true healing can take place. On a cellular level, our bodies respond to our thoughts and attitudes. Whatever we think about our Self, whether it is negative or positive, we send those messages to our body on a cellular level. The mind and body are interconnected, not separate. What our mind conceives, our body believes. The body ultimately responds to the directives that the mind sends it, through years of programming.

Once at a meeting in Santa Barbara, California, someone approached me with a very interesting question. Several of the people in attendance had been drinking the naturally magnetized water for awhile and had shared with other participants their positive results. One of the ladies in attendance, who had been drinking the water for a few months, was obese and had recently experienced an injury to her leg. A very renowned doctor approached me asking about this individual.

'Dr. Ohno, if June is drinking your water, why is she so heavy?"

"Well, there are several reasons why. You have to watch June and listen to her. When she talks she is very negative when she makes any reference to herself. She usually eats the wrong foods. So, even though she drinks the water she offsets the good effect by eating the wrong foods and putting herself down! The water definitely helps her, but if she won't take some responsibility to change her diet and her attitude, the water is not going to benefit like it should."

When we send our body love, it will respond to the vibration of love. So when we are ill, and we respond to the illness with love and compassion, the disease loses its power because we discontinue to feed it with fear. We continue to feed illness as long as we give it power by sending distress and fear to our body. Our cells cannot generate the proper energy, and the immune system will start to shut down when the body is under stress. So if we send fear or stress or anxiety to our cells, then we are not allowing them to produce the antibodies to fight the disease.

Disease is actually Dis-ease, which is an unbalanced state. When we concentrate on appreciating our body and having faith in our cells for their ability to heal themselves, we begin to see improvement. Even though I believe in the water, I know it is limited in its ability to improve health if a person does not honor his or her body or believe in the water.

It is the body's nature to "fight" disease. When someone suffers from cancer, arthritis, or multiple sclerosis, it is natural to have feelings of sadness, fear, anger, helplessness, and apprehension. Our instinct is to fight to get the disease out of our body. But when we feel love for the disease, it loses its power. When we can send love down to the cellular level, we are sending our body healing power. The love we send our body is much more effective than any miracle drug we could hope to discover through research.

How is it possible to love a disease that has inhabited the body? I know this sounds like a strange concept, but it is our negative thoughts and abuse to our body that has caused our disease. When we learn to feel compassion for the disease and understand that it is simply a response to how we have not honored our body in a loving way, we can overcome illness. Understanding certain metaphysical principles and natural laws enables us to rise above our ignorance to a new level of enlightenment.

Do No Harm

This enlightenment releases our ego and centers us within our heart. Once we are centered within our heart, we can enter into a place of love. Love is the greatest force in the universe, and it is love that has the ability to heal everything. It is through love that miracles happen. So when we can find it within our heart to love the unhealed part of us that is crying out for help, we begin to have healing.

Center yourself within your heart ~
Envision a pure white Loving Light

Feel the warmth from the Loving Light and allow yourself to become one with the Love of this Light. Extend the Love in the form of sending Gratitude for all that you are ~ right now!

Continue to feel Love and Appreciation for your body and Miracles will come into your life.

Yoshitaka Ohno, M.D., Ph.D.

Chapter Nine

Sharing My Vision

Shintopia: Mind/Body/Spirit Unity With Nature

Throughout this book I described the special quality of my mother, her mind/body/spirit philosophy. My mother is from a spiritual family, with a long history of spirituality. Her father was a Chief Shinto priest and her younger brother, my uncle, is now Chief Priest of the Kasuga Shrine in Nara, Japan. I have inherited a spiritual nature, which has affected how I view life. My search to become a humanitarian doctor began with a spiritual influence, which has always kept me on the path towards achieving my goals. It is with this introduction that I now explain my vision of following a mind/body/spirit life to achieve a healthier, longer and fuller life.

The name that I created to represent my vision of the mind/body/spirit experience in helping others enjoy a healthier, fuller and longer life is **Shintopia**. I created this term by combining two words, **Shin** and **Utopia**. I learned the values of Shinto, not as a practitioner of a religion, but as a benefactor of what this philosophy offered.

Unlike most people's understanding, Shinto is not a religion, but an ancient philosophy, which when translated means, "To live in harmony with a new heart with all mankind as one with nature." It is humanitarian in concept, but incorporates the spiritual domain. It teaches praise and gratitude for all we are called to do, and recognizes nature as a major force in determining our destinies. Knowledge passed down from centuries of its history has provided important guidelines for many, ancient healing arts, which are popular today. This knowledge was the inspiration for my vision of mind/body/ spirit unity. Utopia is an ideal state. It is also the optimal state of

Do No Harm

health and well-being. Shintopia seemed like the best way to express this concept.

To accept the concept of Shintopia and benefit from what it offers, it is necessary to understand and believe that:

1. There is no single cause for each illness. Disease, like health, is the result of a combination of factors: mind, body, spirit, environment and life choices.

2. There is more than one way for the body to heal. No single approach, practice or treatment can do it all.

3. Healing is not exclusive to medical treatments or pharmaceuticals. With the right approach to using the healing power of mind/body/spirit, in unity with the gifts of nature, health can be restored and maintained.

4. We must take responsibility for our own continuous state of health and well-being.

Inherent in Shintopia are the natural principles and practices of the ancient attitudes, healing philosophies and healing arts, which have been lost and relinquished to modern medicine. On the other hand, my strong background and training in medicine required that I incorporate sound, scientific principles into the development of this vision. The result is bringing humankind and nature together as partners in realizing this vision to help people enjoy a healthier, fuller and longer life.

Its philosophy embraces the universal, natural law of cause and effect. It holds that humans have a responsibility to live with respect for nature and live in communion with all of our earth's natural forces and resources. As we honor and respect ourselves, as we nurture our environment, our gratitude can create action to ensure that the energy of life will create harmony for all life forms.

Yoshitaka Ohno, M.D., Ph.D.

The rewards of accepting this philosophy are achieved through dedication to serve self and humankind. Keeping the unity of mind/body/spirit in balance allows us to focus on striving to maintain this same harmony with nature. I want to share this attitude and commitment with others to offer them the same opportunity to experience the benefits of this Shintopian vision.

Mind/Body/Spirit Unity

The majority of medical scientists follow a common principle regarding health and well-being. **Health and disease are basically determined by states of order and disorder of our body.** Health is more than just the absence of disease. I believe health is a life long journey in discovering the knowledge of how we should live in appreciation of our relationship with nature, and use her gifts with gratitude. It is giving attention to the mind/body/spirit unity that keeps us in balance. It is always showing appreciation and gratitude for the gifts that are given to us when we are open to accept them. Disease is a breakdown of the vital forces that keep our body in balance, therefore, a breakdown of mind/body/spirit unity.

There are three distinct, yet inseparable dimensions to all of us. When these dimensions interact in harmony with each other, we are in a state of optimal health. When any one of these dimensions is not in mutual harmony, the systems of the body become disrupted and break down. A state of stress and anxiety takes over, and we react with alarm, depression, and futility. This creates a biochemical imbalance, depresses the immune system and disrupts metabolism. We become sick.

The disharmony of the physical, or body dimension becomes obvious. Symptoms appear. The body is in distress. But the other dimensions, mind and spirit are not visible, and if we have not learned to be in touch with them, they will affect how our body functions. The mind is the center of our self-perception. A negative attitude creates a negative mental process, which retards healing and balance. The spirit is the vital force that creates our will to focus on a positive attitude, and achieve peace and self-appreciation. A restless spirit creates turmoil within, and leads to attitudes and actions, which destroy the body's balance.

The body, or physical dimension will react to outside therapies and appear healed. But only with a strong belief system, created by the mind and spirit, will the body remain in a state of health. We are not born with the natural ability to maintain a mind/body/spirit harmony. Pressures from daily living and exposure to toxicity in the environment forces the defense systems of the body to struggle to maintain balance. If we have not learned to incorporate the mind and spirit into this healing process, the body will remain vulnerable.

We live and prosper in a mind/body/spirit world, with attitude, action and faith. We focus on consulting with our bodies through mental imaging, meditation, and prayer. We rely on faith in our ability to overcome any health obstacle. We even consult with our bodies on nutritional and exercise needs. We tap into our mind and learn to direct its message system. We tap into our natural instincts that tell us what we need to do and what we need to avoid. This happens when we learn to focus, to direct energy to the source of unbalance in our body.

Nature's Abundant Gift - Water

As we learn to appreciate and live in harmony with nature and focus on our bodies' basic needs, we become aware of nature's most basic gift of life, its water. Saving our environment by establishing attitudes of clean water and preservation of our forests is critical to our survival. Water has been recognized as the source of life since man first became aware of his relationship with nature.

Water has been used as a purification rite and as a source of healing in every civilization since the beginning. The water I discovered in Japan in an area known as Nariwa has been sanctified since early Japanese history. Many legends became popular by those living in this area. One, which dates back to the tenth century, A.D., describes a drought which lasted many years. The people prayed to their gods to send rain. Even though their prayers had been ignored in the past, water began to flow freely from the mountain.

In the thirteenth century, the Emperor, who was terminally ill, sought out a place to die. After being brought to Nariwa, the source of the water from the "magnetic mountain", he was served this water daily by the people and was healed. He brought this water back to his palace in Kyoto and distributed it to his court. All health problems disappeared. This water became known as the "Emperor's Water." A mandate was given that this water was to remain a secret.

After I read about the importance of water in every civilization, I wondered why water was not considered as important today. Everyone thinks water is just H2O; that all water is the same. But all water is not the same. They don't seem to realize how important water is for our body to survive. They don't know that the water most people drink from their faucets is poison.

Then I discovered the naturally magnetized water in Nariwa; the same water I had read about. I did research on how this water affects disease and aging. After spending several years trying to get support for my research, I founded the Ohno Institute on Water and Health, so I could continue my work on discovering causes of and answers to disease and aging problems.

The Ohno Institute was established to learn more about this naturally magnetized water, and study how it supports my vision of a mind/body/spirit humanitarian medicine. The Japanese symbol for "perfect harmony and balance" is Nariwa. This describes the state of our body when it is in mind/body/spirit unity. The source of this water is Nariwa, Japan. This is why I named this special water, Nariwa.

When I established the Ohno Institute on Water and Health, I dedicated it to being a resource center where we could scientifically test the concept of mind/body/spirit unity with nature on improving health. I wanted to share the findings of studies I conducted on the naturally magnetized water I found in Japan. I wanted to make this water available so people could experience how nature provides what our body needs to maintain balance and remain in a state of health. I wanted to learn if Shintopia could help people trapped in chronic illness gain a greater sense of self, a greater appreciation of life, and a freedom from stress and despair, which leads to illness.

Because this Institute is not owned or controlled by any large organization or institution with a governing body that could set restrictive policies, I have the freedom to provide service to anyone seeking answers to health and aging problems. I have the luxury of consulting with the best minds in both conventional and alternative medicine. I have become both student and teacher. I must work extra hard to argue my philosophy and vision. But I work with gratitude for those who have helped me develop and communicate my vision, as well as to those who have helped me collect evidence to explain mind/body/spirit unity in clarifying this vision.

The Shintopian Concept of Mind/Body/Spirit Unity

This Shintopian vision is actually a vision of hope that is given by understanding certain basic principles of life enhancement. As we evolve through the events of our life, new lessons are always presenting themselves for our continuation of growth. As long as we are able to focus on the present moment and allow ourselves to concentrate on the here and now, we can teach ourselves to tune into and develop basic principles that enhance our world. The more we learn to develop and exercise these basic principles into our daily life, the better our life becomes. The mind/body/spirit concept of Shintopia encompasses the basic principles of invisible energy, balance, personal responsibility, contribution, self-love and gratitude, which enhances the Shintopian effect.

Yoshitaka Ohno, M.D., Ph.D.

Learning how to recognize and how to use the *invisible energy* that is always present and helping to direct our decisions will keep us on line with our true path. Exercising our *personal responsibility* ultimately brings us in control with our own self-empowerment. Through the act of *contribution*, we connect with a fundamental need from the deepest part of our being to selflessly give of our heart. By discovering how to establish internal *balance* we learn how to maintain an equilibrium that enhances our ability to make rightful decisions. And the greatest principle of all, *self-love*, is the highest form of expression we can give back to honor our soul to bring fulfillment into our life. This is expressed as *gratitude* in all that is given to us.

This is what the concept of Shintopia is about. My dream is to build a center for Mind/Body/Spirit Medicine where Shintopia will eventually be practiced. But I have come to realize that each person *is his/her own Health and Healing Center*. People are responsible for their health and well being by their thoughts and actions, and have the innate ability to heal and remain healthy. And so it is that a Shintopian vision is synonymous with the concept of hope, because without hope, faith cannot be exercised. It takes only a small amount of faith to turn our world around into a harmonious expression of life.

Invisible Energy - Hidden But Always Present

Invisible energy is a loving and spiritual guidance that is connected from the all knowing, universal mind. This loving and gentle guidance communicates to us through our senses, our intuition, and our ability to 'tune in' to a quiet deeper knowing that is felt on a spiritual level. However, most people do not realize the importance of this energy because they have a highly developed ego, which associates with the outer world and not the inner world. Sometimes we place our value on gaining financial success, or on relationship issues, or obtaining material possessions.

Do No Harm

When all of our concentration is centered on how our life is progressing, it is difficult to be still and listen to the subtle messages that are always present and available for our betterment. The person we want to be or want to become gets in the way of our focus. Seldom do we recognize the wonderful hidden energy that is waiting to give us insight and understanding about our life. If we concentrate on the ego and allow it to inhabit our world, it will be too difficult to recognize the guidance of invisible energy when it appears before us.

"Throw away the controlling ego and make your mind naked.
You will definitely feel the invisible energy when
Your mind is free to be receptive."

The more we develop ego, the less we are able to receive the messages delivered from the invisible energy. The ego does not have to be *completely* abandoned, because a healthy ego is necessary for keeping our balance. However, when we can recognize that we do not have to abandon the ego, but simply not allow it to manipulate our life, then we can ease into allowing the intuitive invisible energy to help guide us. When we connect with and follow the urgings that feel right with our heart, then we are allowing invisible energy to work in our lives.

Sometimes it is not until years have passed that we can look back on our life to see how the pieces of the puzzle have come together. While we are in the middle of a life event, fear and apprehension often clouds our vision so that we do not see the overall view. But nearly always, when we review our life we can see why certain things took place and how the direction of our lives was forever changed. The secret is to gain the insight and self-trust *during* the moment in our life when these changes are taking place. This is when invisible energy becomes so valuable.

Recognizing Invisible Energy

Yoshitaka Ohno, M.D., Ph.D.

The best way to know that you are following your highest guidance is by listening to your heart and what feels right to you. Becoming quiet and still to tune in to your true feelings is essential when linking with the energy of the higher mind. When joy is connected with the decisions you are making, then you are always doing what is in your best interest. If hesitation, concern, fear or worry is connected with the decisions you are making, then realignment will eventually need to be addressed. Negativity is never part of the equation for what is in your best interest. *"Always go with your first instinct."* We have heard this phrase repeated so many times probably because it is so true!

Personal Responsibility

With enlightenment comes responsibility

As we gain an understanding of the power of invisible energy and how to use it for our betterment, a degree of personal responsibility becomes activated. When we treat our body or our life as though we do not honor our greater good, we eventually create discomfort in our world. The law of cause and effect responds to our thoughts and actions; and it is only a matter of time before the transference of this energy manifests itself into our life.

The events of our life are not pre-programmed or predetermined, leaving us to be swept along through life feeling detached and useless. Rather, we are always in control of the progressive events by our active participation through the decisions we make every moment of every day. We gain an active control by utilizing our personal responsibility to recognize and make healthy decisions that enhance our greater good.

Becoming responsible for our actions awards us with a wonderful feeling of self-empowerment! Have you ever been determined to do something important in your life to the extent

Do No Harm

that you've placed all of your focus on your goal? Have you felt the exhilaration of accomplishment for something you believed in? There is a saying that goes, *"True freedom is derived directly from your personal degree of responsibility."* There is a great deal of truth to this message. The more we can become responsible for our actions, the more freedom we gain in our lives.

Few situations in life are as gratifying as Self-Empowerment when you have used it toward your greater good!

Astronauts have recognized the unique beauty of the earth from their view thousands of miles away. Many astronauts have received spiritual insights and experiences after joining with the stars and gaining an appreciation for what our planet offers. Even though there are so many planets in our solar system, earth is very special because it is the only planet with the miracle of life. Earth is perfectly positioned in relation to the sun, which creates the perfect venue for life. Earth is also made up of 70% water and it is the water that maintains the harmonious balance for our climate.

Our body also requires balance and circulation, and the human body also consists of 70% water. Oriental medicine has the philosophy that the human body and the universe are the same. It is essential that the water on earth be uncontaminated in order for life on our planet to continue. Our health is directly dependent upon the quality of our water consumption.

When our bodies are unhealthy our minds are not in a clear state. When our bodies are sick we are preoccupied with concern for our health. Fear and worry become our focus because we want to bring our body back to a state of wellness. These negative associations create emotional imbalance, which affects the decisions we make.

Honoring our minds and bodies with healthy food and water is our personal responsibility. When we ignore the importance of taking care of our body we are not honoring our greater good.

Yoshitaka Ohno, M.D., Ph.D.

When our minds are sending us messages that we are not treating ourselves in the best manner possible, we are not in a state of mental balance.

Balance and Emotional Equilibrium

The balance between the mind, body and
spirit are all connected~
The way we nurture one affects the health of the three.

The times I have been able to make the decisions with the greatest clarity for rightful action are the times I have been emotionally balanced. There is something to be said about emotional equilibrium that cultivates inner wisdom. When tuning in to receive the invisible energy of intuition, becoming still and quiet is essential.

Emotions are a vital part of being human. One of the gifts we have in our human experience is to *feel* and experience the emotions of our human nature. Emotions are the results of our thoughts, and they are meant to be expressed and released. But once released, allow the emotion to let go, especially if it is a feeling of fear, guilt, anger or sadness. Decisions that are made in our best interest are ones made when we are mentally relaxed and balanced, not when we are angry or upset.

Contribution - The Act of Selfless Giving

Contribution is a vital component of human nature that allows us to give a part of ourselves to humanity. Giving from one's heart with no strings attached is one of the most important gifts we can give back to our self.

"As you give - so shall you receive".

People who have become successful and have accomplished everything they have set out to do often feel an indescribable emptiness. So they continue to search for another triumph to help them become complete. And yet they still feel void of fulfillment. Unless the act of contribution is aligned with their life purpose they will continue to experience the uneasy feeling of emptiness.

When you give from your heart and experience bringing joy into someone's life, there is nothing that feeds the soul more. There is a sense of completeness that overwhelms our true nature when we administer serving another person or devote ourselves to a cause we believe in. The greatest fulfillment I receive is when I have helped to give someone a sense of hope. Hope to know that they can once again become healthy and happy. Hope to know that another person truly cares about their needs. Hope to know that they are not alone. Hope to know that they also have ability to give hope to another person in need.

The beautiful thing about contribution is that it doesn't have to cost anything. Selfless acts of kindness can be as simple as giving a smile or a word of encouragement. I often receive intuitive messages telling me to say something kind to a complete stranger. In the matter of a few precious moments you can turn the course of a person's day around just by following your inner urge to extend a simple act of kindness.

When you freely give of yourself you open up your heart. And when your heart becomes open you create expansion in your life to receive good. What you give you ultimately receive back because what goes around comes around. But it is imperative to give without looking for what you can receive in return. If you give only for what you will gain out of it, the gift of contribution has lost its true meaning. You may create the scenario of people taking advantage of your 'good nature' and you will wonder why this happens to you. But when you give with absolutely no strings attached, then you will receive appreciation from the universe for your warm and kind heart. Your heart and spirit expand to receive the energy from your gift of contribution.

Yoshitaka Ohno, M.D., Ph.D.

Self-Love - Appreciation for Our Life

Unconditional love for our bodies and for the gift of our passage is what feeds our spirit and gives us life force. This is unconditional love for the state of our life as it is in the here and the now. No matter what you look like, how much you weigh, how much money you currently make or what transition you are evolving through at the given moment, love your Self just as you are.

When we feed love to our mind, body and soul, our spirit responds and heals our life. As we are continually in the process of wanting to 'change' ourselves for the better, it is natural to be critical of our current conditions. However, it is in sending love and compassion to our current condition that we open the universal energy to create positive change in our lives.

Have you ever really shown appreciation and gratitude to your body? Think of all the organs that compose your body. Become aware of your liver, your heart, your stomach, your brain, your mouth, your eyes, and so on. Your body has worked for you unconditionally for all of the years you have lived. Unless you have experienced an illness or accident that has caused part of your body to stop functioning, you still have a supporting and loving body housing your spirit as you continue your life on the planet. Send appreciation to your body and watch it respond!

Give appreciation to your body by taking good care of it. Feed it healthy foods and give it proper exercise and sleep. Fuel it with inspiration and knowledge that keeps your mind growing and expanding. Send appreciation for the loving way your body works for you day in and day out, without a break, continually working to keep you alive. If we stop for a moment to imagine all of our body functions and feel the love our body has for us, we gain a deep love for the gift we have been given. And when we are ill, sending love to the illness that is in our body is the best way to release the illness and let it leave our body. When we hate the disease and react in a combative manner, we are also

Do No Harm

hating our bodies and fighting against our own state of health. Giving appreciation opens up your heart and expands your vibrational energy.

Sending appreciation and love to where you are in your life is the most effective way of creating a more successful and better future for your Self. Today we are planting the seeds for our tomorrow. If we can begin to feel the joy for our life in the present moment, we are planting the seeds to generate a joyous future. If we hate our life, our spouse, our job, our home, and our life in general, we are sending an unloving part of ourselves to greet us in the future. Our true power to appreciate is in the present moment; it is in the present moment that we have the ability to alter the direction of our life.

Genuine self-love is the greatest gift you will ever give your soul. It is amazing to watch how your life changes for the better when you bring love into all of the situations in your world. You release blocks of negativity that free you to be open and aware to listen to the messages from a loving invisible energy that is patiently waiting to guide you. You enter into a true sense of personal responsibility. Because you feel so much love, you automatically want to do what is best for your life. You ease into balance because you are happier and more centered on a soul level. You feel a true need to contribute often to people and causes in need. You want to share your love because it feeds back to you.

Enthusiasm is very contagious ~
It is an important and joyous component to our nature.

I know that it has been because of the lessons I have learned and the choices I have made that eventually led me to my vision. The decisions I've made have often been very difficult because I was going against the normal flow. I had the courage to declare my individual course and I have often experienced an alienation and detachment from society. But I have always been able to live with my decisions even through difficult times. This is

Yoshitaka Ohno, M.D., Ph.D.

because I have been able to maintain the integrity of my personal belief system. I know that because of this attitude, I was able to plan and build the Ohno Institute and keep it going, despite many difficulties in keeping it moving forward.

The only person you ever have to answer to is your <u>Self</u>
To your own Self, be true!

I have been very blessed to have a strong family foundation that has given me immeasurable love and encouragement. My mother Yoshiko, and my wife, Akiko, have always stood close by my side with their undying faith in me. This everlasting faith has aided in giving me a tremendous amount of courage to follow my heart instead of being drawn into what the masses were doing. I realize that not everyone has a strong family support system that enables him or her to find strength when times are difficult. I know that it is easier to force yourself into decisions that do not follow your inner desires when you are overwhelmed by intimidation. Many people are not following the desires that come from their hearts because of fear. People fear they will become outcasts from society, or they will not be able to provide for themselves if they walk to the beat of their own drum.

When we listen to and trust our personal truth, we are being guided by a loving, invisible energy that is watching over us and encouraging our growth. This is when we provide ourselves with our own personal support system. Regardless of weak personal and family relationships, there is only *one* person to whom we truly need to answer, our Self. No matter how long we are given the privilege to live, we will always be living with the person we presently are and the person we are in the process of becoming.

The struggle, agonies and challenges I have experienced have gradually led me to recognize my destiny. I know that I have a need to spread happiness by giving hope to mankind. I have always had a gift of having a compassionate voice and

Do No Harm

mannerism to which people react. My patients have often remarked that they feel a natural healing energy as they listen to my voice and are affected by my calming vibration. I also believe that discovering and giving naturally magnetized water to people has also given me a way of making a true contribution to humanity. Every time I help someone by giving them this water to improve their health, I am immediately energized with excitement and joy. I feel alive with a wonderful enthusiasm for the hope I know I have been able to give, because hope is healing and can make a tremendous difference in someone's life.

The truth of my Shintopian vision of mind/body/spirit unity with nature is fueled by the energy from the natural forces of universe, Nariwa water, and the passion that drives me. The evidence which supports this truth will be gathered from my continuous effort to learn more about how our bodies respond to the healing effects of Nariwa water through research at the Ohno Institute. Everyone is invited to share this vision and experience a healthier, longer, and fuller life.

Yoshitaka Ohno, M.D., Ph.D.

About the Author

Yoshitaka Ohno, M.D., Ph.D.,
Founder and President
Ohno Institute on Water and Health

Dr. Ohno is a native of Osaka, Japan, where he received his education and training in medicine and neuropathology. Early in his medical career, he began searching for ways to stop the suffering of his patients with diseases that could not be treated successfully by standard medicine, and thus had to be managed with multiple drugs. He began to realize that the side effects of these drugs were creating serious chronic problems, as well as increasing the body's deterioration. After extensive study he became convinced that the condition of the body's water was directly related to the state of the body's health.

After leaving his medical practice, he continued his studies but found that the Japanese medical community was not placing much emphasis on chronic diseases found commonly among the aging population. He decided to enter the United States and accept a position at AMC Hospital in Denver, Colorado, where he could continue his research in geriatric pathology, including MRI studies on the relationship of water and cellular degeneration. His work led him to investigate the neuropathology of Alzheimer's disease. As a result of his work, he received the *Community Leadership Award* from the Colorado Alzheimer's Association in 1987, and the *Humanitarian Award* from the Alzheimer's Disease International in 1993.

After returning to Japan in 1990, he discovered a naturally magnetized water that was being used by a prominent physician to treat serious, life-threatening diseases. As these patients recovered, Dr. Ohno became convinced that this water was unique. He pursued numerous clinical studies with this water, both in Japan and the United States. In 1998, Dr. Ohno founded the Ohno Institute on Water and Health, a non-profit research and education center for studying the effect of naturally magnetized water on health and aging. He has been requested as a speaker at several health conferences and has published several articles in professional journals on his findings.

Dr. Ohno resides with his wife and three children in Chagrin Falls, Ohio.

Printed in the United States
2327